Agency, Heal
Surv
The Ecopolitics of Rival
Psychologies

Caroline New

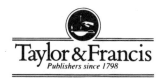

Taylor & Francis
Publishers since 1798

UK   Taylor & Francis Ltd, 1 Gunpowder Square, London EC4A 3DE
USA   Taylor & Francis Inc., 1900 Frost Road, Suite 101, Bristol, PA 19007

First published 1996

**A Catalogue Record for this book is available from the British
Library**

ISBN 0 7484 0246 2
ISBN 0 7484 0247 0 (pbk)

**Library of Congress Cataloging-in-Publication Data are available on
request**

Typeset in 10/12 pt Times
by Graphicraft Typesetters Limited, Hong Kong

Printed in Great Britain by SRP Ltd., Exeter

Contents

Acknowledgments   viii

Chapter 1   Introduction   1
Moments of conception   1
Contending philosophies: Contending anxieties   3
Critical realism   6
The project of the book   8

Chapter 2   Starting points   12
What is?   12
What should be?   14
What can be? Structures   16
What can be? Human capacities   18
Can human beings change society?   20
Deliberate social change   23
Motivation and the need for psychology   25

Chapter 3   Conflicting concepts of health   29
Agency, health and human capacities   29
The coming of aetiology and the mind/body split   31
Mental health and 'illness': The limits of relativism   35
Positive health versus health as normal functioning   37
Conclusion   42

Chapter 4   Freud and the inevitability of discontent   46
Introduction   46
The first Freud: The trauma or seduction theory   48
The second Freud: Infantile sexuality and psychic reality   52
The aetiological role of social structures   54
Mental health in the dynamic theory   57
The death instinct and the origins of morality   58
Civilization and renunciation   60

Psychological health: The view from ego-psychology   62
Psychic processes and social structures   66

Chapter 5   Melanie Klein: A social emotion   70
Introduction   70
The baby, its inner life and the external world   73
Psychic structures, social structures   76
What is psychological health?   80
Conclusion   84

Chapter 6   Jacques Lacan: Exposing the myth of agency   87
Introduction   87
Early work: From alienation to Oedipus   91
Penis and phallus   92
Desire: A human natural capacity   95
What is psychological health?   96
Psychic structures, social structures?   99
Political possibilities: Lacan and others   101

Chapter 7   Humanistic psychology: Saved by synergy   103
Introduction   103
Human nature and the real self   106
Needs and the vicissitudes of the self   109
What is psychological health?   111
Psychic structures, social structures   113

Chapter 8   Four radical approaches   119
Introduction: Lines of demarcation   119
Power, knowledge and the aim of therapy   124
Oppression is bad for your health   130
Beyond the deficit model   134
Conclusion   141

Chapter 9   Conclusion: If humanly possible   143
Four necessary conditions for radical change   143
The ecopolitics of rival psychologies   144
    Freud and ego-psychology   145
    Klein and the Kleinians   146
    Humanistic psychologies   147
    Radicals   149
Embryonic green psychologies   151
    Environmentalism   151
    Social ecology   152

Contents

Deep ecology   154
Ecofeminism   157
Conclusion   159

Notes   168
References   171
Index   183

Acknowledgments

This work has been eight years in the making and more people have assisted me with it than I can possibly acknowledge. Friends who managed to convince me that they look forward to reading the published book, or simply that they thought the work important, have made a big difference. They know who they are. More formally I want to thank the following, who read individual chapters in draft and gave me their comments: Kate Barrows, Paul Barrows, Rosie Brennan, Fiona Gardiner, Keith Graham, Francis Roberts, Janet Sayers, Sean Sayers, Jem Thomas and Andrew Woodfield.

Discussions with many people have helped my work. In particular I remember the generosity of Gloria Babicker, Peter Baehr, Chris Bertram, Roy Bhaskar, Jean Briggs, Andrew Collier, Sheila Ernst, Margaret Green, David Hirschman, Ursula Kelly, Gary Kinsman, Ruth Levitas, John Lovering, John Morissey, Adam Morton, Barbara Neis, Maureen Ramsey, Joanna Ryan and Will Wright. Thanks also to the Red-Green Study Group, whose discussions have been important for their lack of sectarianism as well as for their content; to the participants in the Realism and the Human Sciences conferences, and also those at the Free Associations conferences on Psychoanalysis and the Public Sphere. I have appreciated consistent and friendly support from my colleagues at Bath College of Higher Education; and the encouragement, confidence and patience of my family. Thanks to the skilled practitioners who have helped to minimize the various physical difficulties that have beset me and delayed the work: Paul Baker, Ali Burrows, John Leah, Eli Melgaard and Diane Tanner; and to Brian Bocking and John Cooper who rescued my notes from the maw of the computer. Above all, thanks to those who read the entire work and commented on it: Ted Benton, Jo Campling, Norman Freeman, Linda Martin, and especially Paul Hoggett for his enthusiastic long-term encouragement and creative help.

Chapter 1

Introduction

Moments of conception

One of several moments of this book's conception took place in a classroom in Newfoundland in the early 1980s. I was teaching a course on 'Classical Social Theory' in Memorial University's summer school. To illustrate a point about Marx, I showed the students a film on the increase in productivity in the fishing industry. Newfoundland and Labrador is Canada's easternmost province, a relatively under-developed region of high unemployment. Newfoundland itself is an enormous rocky island, so scattered with lakes and pools that it looks lacy from the air. Stunted conifers cover its infertile soil. Beyond its rocky coast swim not only whales, but schools of cod, and capelin, a sardine-like fish on which both cod and whales feed. Every summer the beaches are strewn with the stinking corpses of the male capelin, which die after breeding. And every summer huge Japanese ships dock in St John's harbour, their hulls stuffed with the bodies of the female capelin, prized for their roe. Once upon a time the inshore fishermen in the 'outports' could make a living by fishing as long as the seas weren't frozen. In the 1980s they tended to work ten weeks a year, to entitle them to unemployment pay for the rest of the year. Only the trawlers, the deepsea fishers who pull up everything, could reach the remaining cod. Now, in the 1990s, there is a moratorium on fishing.

In the classroom, the whirring images of these trawlers showed their decks covered continuously, sometimes 24 hours a day, with squirming silver fish end-lessly taken from the deeps. Here was Newfoundland's wealth, through that in-creased productivity of which both Marxists and capitalist apologists approved, being squandered at source. Even I, a long-time believer in economic progress, was forcibly struck by the reality of the finitude of resources and the likelihood of a relationship between that greedy plunder and the undeniable evidence – outside the classroom – of Newfoundland's dying, hostage economy.

By the time of this unpleasant and urgent realization, an earlier and long-drawn out moment of conception had already occurred. In the first half of the 1970s I was first an Althusserian intellectual and then a socialist feminist activist. In Althusserian circles I met others who, like me, took the basic truth of psychoana-lysis for granted. Yet, unlike me, most of my highly theoreticist comrades seemed totally uninterested in things personal or psychological. For them the subject was an illusory construction, yet they hailed psychoanalysis (in the abstract) as scientific. What also came to puzzle me was the structuralist rejection, in the name of anti-empiricism, of any causal role for subjective experience. How could this be reconciled with our active political aims and affiliations? This puzzlement came to a head when I had my first baby. Various aspects of women's position in society which I had previously 'known' hit me with the force of a sledgehammer and I could not account for the power of this new way of knowing. Some years later I was still distancing myself – but now as a socialist feminist – from those parts of the women's liberation movement which extolled women's experience as the unproblematic source of knowledge. At that period I used to wonder to what extent various psychoanalytic theories were really compatible with feminist aims. I still do. The intellectual acceptance of psychoanalytic theory by non-clinicians often remains abstract, unrelated to political and theoretical tenets and aims with which it may actually be inconsistent.

My two emerging questions were: 'How can human societies become both sustainable and just?' and 'What does the human mind have to be like, if socialist and feminist aims are to be achievable?' or, coming at it from another angle: 'What are the political implications of psychoanalysis and other theories of human subjectivity?' The long history of my own refusal to think about the need for sustainability served to underline the point that rationalist notions of political consciousness were extraordinarily naïve.

Maybe social transformation *can* be brought about by people deliberately and collectively acting in ways they have reason to believe will be transformative. If so, it does not follow that they will take such action because they have read a leaflet or gone to a public meeting setting out 'the facts'. Generations of political thought did not seem to have progressed far beyond this model. Both social theorists and activists needed psychological theory, I came to believe, but needed to approach it cautiously and critically because of the occupational hazard of its own creators, the tendency to treat the subject as presocial (Henriques *et al.*, 1984). As a materialist, and therefore a philosophical realist, I was assuming that the world held answers to my questions, even if these answers were never vouchsafed to me. (Of course, the answers might be of the Wittgensteinian sort which deconstruct the question and the sense of puzzlement with it.) I assumed (and still assume) that the human mind has certain capacities, certain developmental tendencies, which permit certain social possibilities and forbid others; and that we can come to know these structures, capacities and tendencies through theorizing their effects. I assumed that approaching such questions from the direction of the *social* – both what psychological theorizing presupposes about the social and what it implies about the social – would begin to put flesh on the bare bones of the concept of agency. I had not really taken on board poststructuralist and postmodernist scepticism about the subject, about agency and about knowledge. A dialogue with postmodernism is the third of the formative moments of this book.

In one of the many conversations that composed this dialogue a friend and I grew tired of the obstinate counterposition of concepts and arguments that slid past each other without really engaging. Instead, she asked me why I so disliked poststructuralism, especially its relativism and scepticism about reality outside of discourse. I replied that it seemed to lead to nihilism and political cynicism or self-deception. If I were really to accept its rejection of the possibility of knowledge, I would feel I was going mad. But why did she, a working-class feminist, hold to it so strongly? Because, she said, her inner fragmentation felt so extreme that only a theory that articulated it could prevent her feeling *she* was going mad. For a while there was not much more either of us could say. I began to see that philosophical disputes may be reflections of contending anxieties.

Contending philosophies: Contending anxieties

Postmodernists rightly insist that knowledge is always partial and always situated. For me, this indicates the nature of the foundations of knowledge rather than undermining them. The autobiographical history of ideas above is offered in a postmodern spirit by a writer – a middle-class, middle-aged, white, English, female writer – who is intellectually and politically committed to the Enlightenment ideal of human emancipation. I am uncomfortable with Habermas' phrase 'the project of modernity' to summarize this commitment, because I find 'modernity' too broad and too tendentious a concept. Wherever we draw its boundaries, modernity spawned many and inconsistent projects, including those firmly opposed to emancipation. Habermas also describes this project as aiming to bring society, *like nature*, under control for the emancipation of humankind generally (1983, p. 9). Here I would agree with postmodern critics that what we do *not* need, and what is arguably behind the disastrous poverty of Africa today, is the attempt to control society *in the way* industrialized nations have attempted to control nature. How we control society, and who 'we' are, remain unanswered for the present, but my starting point is that we must do so in order to prevent continuing, even increasing human suffering and eventual social extinction. This, then, is the source of my anxiety and of my hope.

Following Foucault (1980, p. 131), many postmodernists find the very epistemology of modernity, the insistence on the distinction between Truth and Rhetoric, inherently authoritarian. For some, characterizations of social reality are rationalizations of 'aspirations for social authority' (Seidman, 1992, p. 55). Knowledge is always situated and relative, never universal; it can have no sure foundations. The only philosophically (and therefore politically) defensible route open to postmodernists interested in social theory is as providers of 'contextualized local narratives' (op. cit., p. 50). 'People do not suffer as members of categories, but in specific times and places ... An ironic general social theory, a postmodern social theory, requires the easy sacrifice of a modernist commitment to a reality that cannot be confirmed' (Lemert, 1992, p. 41). For these thinkers, the Marxist notions of ideology and false consciousness, the feminist conviction that women are everywhere oppressed, whether or not they describe themselves as such, simply constitute further evidence for the postmodern belief 'that the Enlightenment project was doomed to turn against itself and transform the quest for human emancipation into a system of universal oppression in the name of human liberation' (Harvey, 1990, p. 13).

The danger, from a postmodern standpoint, lies in essentialism and universals, in refusing to relativize. The postmodern anxiety is that emancipationists are engaged in telling other people what they experience and what is good for them. Pretending to have privileged access to objective knowledge – the 'view from nowhere' (Haraway, 1991) – they are actually bidding for domination. Bauman (1989), for instance, believes that emancipatory practice, which insists on the validity of universal values and categories, cannot ever be genuinely emancipatory from the viewpoint of those whose own experiences, categories and values have been subordinated to the supposedly 'universal' and 'objective' ones of the 'liberators'. He argues that the greatest cruelties and disasters of modern history result from the emancipatory 'project of modernity'. For him, social engineering is entirely discredited (1989, p. 4); the Holocaust can only be understood in its normality, as a climax of instrumental rationality (op. cit., ch. 4); while socialism 'put modernity to its ultimate test. The failure was as ultimate as the test itself' (Bauman, 1990, p. 23). From this point of view the project of emancipation is no more or less than the 'will to power'. The only safe course, from this point of view, is to reject the 'totalitarian myth of the Ideal City' (Laclau and Mouffe, 1985, p. 190) and to give up global aspirations other than those for diversity, tolerance and pluralism.

Epistemologically there is something puzzling about this preference for the local. People suffer in specific times and places, true, but very frequently *because* they are members of certain social categories. So why this emphasis on the local as the only admissible form of knowledge claims on the one hand and the site of 'safe' (i.e. non-oppressive) politics on the other? First, 'local narratives' admit to their origins, are contextualized in this sense. Their validity, or lack of it, depends on their status within the local discourses within which their stories are told. If we, as social scientists, want to provide a gloss on the stories the locals tell, we can at least refer it back to their own versions and respectfully offer it them as potentially useful knowledge (Bauman, 1989a, p. 50). But this attempt to reconcile the practice of social science with postmodern scruples cannot hold water. For local narratives inevitably universalize and make wider claims, or at least do so implicitly by ruling out certain ways of thinking. Social scientists cannot push the cup of meta-judgement from their lips. As Sayer says: 'We can't simply refuse to make *any* evaluation, negative or positive, because unless we decide whether the actors' own explanations of their actions are right, we cannot decide what explanation to choose ourselves' (1992, p. 40). The postmodern insistence that relativism is a necessity of the current epoch is itself, as many have pointed out, a universalizing claim.

Even if there is no good *philosophical* reason for privileging 'local' knowledge, might there not be good *political* reasons for both acting and thinking locally rather than globally? Foucault's insistence on the ubiquity and dispersion of power necessarily suggested a micro-politics. In the case of say, Baudrillard, this becomes nihilistic, while in some cases the 'new pluralism' is not readily distinguishable from the old. However, not all postmodern thinkers reject political action on an international scale. Laclau and Mouffe argue for 'radical democracy', in which decisions are made 'from below' on the basis of many communities and identities, 'breaking with the provincial myth of the "universal class . . ." there is no *a priori* centrality determined at the level of structure, simply because there is no rational foundation of History' (Laclau and Mouffe, 1985, p. 77).

Aaronowitz (1988), who suspects that their 'radical democracy' assumes some universal values and is therefore not as postmodern as they claim, argues for a process of deconstructing 'given' political categories to result in an ever more complex pluralist paradigm, in which new social movements speak 'a language of localism and regionalism, a discourse that . . . addresses power itself as an antagonist' (Aaronowitz, 1988, p. 61). Despite his strictures to Laclau and Mouffe, he nowhere explains *why* power is always to be opposed, using the word 'progressive' as if its meaning were unproblematic.

These confusions occur because there are two major strands in postmodern thinking. One is extreme anti-foundationalism of the sort that sees the world as constructed in language: 'outside of any discursive contexts objects *do not have* being; they only have *existence*' (Laclau and Mouffe, 1987, p. 85). Combined with Foucault's Nietzschean view of power, this is an idealism that effectively makes politics entirely subjective and prohibits rational argument about it. The other strand is a periodization thesis which points out the specific features of the current epoch and the inadequacy of Marxist and other modern sociological characterizations of it (although in fact it is very dependent on them for many of its key concepts). This, essentially realist, position is often combined with an essentially universalist ethical rejection of domination and a valorization of autonomy, self-determination, tolerance and diversity.

This strand of postmodern thinking is, I believe, inconsistent with the first strand's rejection of ontological realism and values of universal scope. Yet they are frequently held by the same people and even put forward in the same works (e.g. Beck, 1992; Laclau and Mouffe, 1987; Bauman, 1989). I suspect that the postmodern anxiety about discursive domination, and about the oppressive potential of 'emancipatory' practices, would be better converted into an attitude of caution and insistence on continuous critique (cf. Isaac, 1990). If allowed to stifle political activity, confine it to micro-politics or resign it to cynicism, it prepares the ground for the emergence of the other anxiety, the one that haunts emancipationists. Perhaps the squirmings of Laclau and Mouffe, for instance, are merely attempts to navigate an impossible path between the Scylla and Charybdis of these two awful visions.

The emancipationist anxiety comes from the secular perception of human beings as uniquely self-conscious and alone in a universe we cannot control, powerless in the face of the unintended consequences of our own social practices. This has a new poignancy in the late-twentieth century, when, in Giddens' words, humanity is riding a juggernaut, 'a runaway engine of enormous power which, collectively as human beings, we can drive to some extent but which also threatens to rush out of our control and which could rend itself asunder' (1990, p. 139). Emancipationists might agree with Bauman that the Gulag and the Holocaust can only be understood in their normality, in their continuity with periods and practices that are taken for granted rather than denounced and represented as alien. Nevertheless, they would want to explain these specific oppressive practices in terms of particular and complex historical causes, rather than as the inevitable result of Utopian endeavours or a universal, essentialist 'will to power'. For emancipationists, postmodern politics amount to an uneasy choice between a sentimental celebration of cut-throat diversity, an espousal of *laissez-faire* capitalism dressed up as a new pluralism, or a neo-anarchist commitment to resistance that eschews any alternative forms of power. Such offerings weigh light indeed when balanced against the fear of social and physical extinction.

Postmodernists and emancipationists may well share various emotions: anger, repugnance and fear evoked by social structures which necessitate and justify human suffering; fear especially of social and environmental degradation and death. These can become fuel for emancipatory projects when combined with 'Utopian' beliefs about the possibility of other ways of living, immanent in existing structures, and an 'objective' concept of oppression. To be coherent, the concept of emancipation requires one of oppression, and the justification of projects of emancipation depends on being able to offer objective indices of oppression. We must be able to say that slavery is wrong, even if slaves appear to accept it.

I shall argue in Chapters 1 and 2 that such emancipatory critique is most powerfully rooted in conceptions of human nature, especially human needs, and in notions of positive health. Philosophically, such conceptions require us to be realists, claiming that it is possible to identify and theorize the human capacities which underlie social life and partially determine the range of its possible forms. For these purposes, the most useful recent 'underlabouring' for the human sciences has been done by critical realists such as Bhaskar, Benton, Soper, Collier, Rustin and others. I use and build on this approach in this book.

Critical realism

Critical realism (sometimes called 'transcendental' or 'scientific' realism) assumes that:

1 At any one moment reality exists independent of human descriptions of it, though it may, the next moment, be affected by such descriptions. (The social world is particularly so affected, but the relationship is *causal* rather than *reductive*, cf. Giddens (1990, p. 43)). The universe existed and had certain characteristics before there were any human beings around to perceive them, and may do so again. Its being 'experienced or experienci-able' is not an 'essential property of the world' but an 'accidental property of some things' (Bhaskar, 1975, p. 28) – for some other things may exist which human beings are incapable of experiencing.

2   We can know what the world is like, though our knowledge is always fallible and incomplete (Sayer, 1992, p. 79; Giddens, 1990, p. 47). Knowledge is always partial and a mere stage in an ongoing process which is by no means obliged to be unidirectional. However, in making a statement about social reality I need not be laying claim to special access to the view from everywhere, but contributing to its formulation by insisting on the view from where I sit. I may be claiming that a certain position (always to some extent arrived at through a collective process) makes sense from *anywhere*. Knowledge is not only reached and assessed within the ways of conceptualizing sometimes called 'discourses' or, more narrowly, 'language-games'; it is also reached as a result of their overlap and mutual influence, and assessed in terms of its adequacy as a guide to practice (Sayer, 1992). This is possible precisely because the world exists outside of the meanings humans use to represent and grasp it and sometimes reminds us, gently or abruptly, when those meanings are misleading.

To non-philosophers these statements may seem obvious or obscure. They are highly relevant, though, to current disputes. The point is that in their extreme forms, poststructuralism and postmodernism tend to espouse the position that the world is actually *given shape* by human descriptions of it. Not just that we can describe in many possible ways, usefully or ineffectually, structures that already exist and that are therefore part of the causal preconditions of our conceptualizing. No, rather that our conceptualizing itself gives form to the formless (Foucault, 1970, p. xx). This is the ontology that refuses to distinguish between science and myth. If there is no world outside of discourse, our concepts are themselves robbed of their causal purchase on the world. 'Causing' (i.e. constructing) everything, by the same token they cause nothing. They become impotent, wheels which turn without connecting with anything. The aim of understanding society better in order to bring about desired social purposes becomes otiose. This position – let us call it P1 – of 'discourse reductionism' is quite incompatible with (1) above.

Second, many postmodernists take the related position – call it P2 – that the concept of knowledge makes sense only in relation to particular discursive contexts. We have therefore no valid way of judging *between* different theoretical discourses and the knowledges they produce. If you hold P1, you have to hold P2, because if to know is to create a world rather than to discover one, the only criteria for validity must be internal to the process of creation. But it is possible not to hold P1, or to limit its application to the social world, and still to agree with at least the first part of P2. Critical realists *would* hold to what Bhaskar calls 'epistemic relativism', 'which asserts that all beliefs are socially produced, so that all knowledge is transient, and neither truth-values nor criteria of rationality exist outside historical time' (Bhaskar, 1975, p. 57).

Although the world is objectively structured, human knowledge of these structures is always partial and relative to our experiences, perspectives and purposes. What critical realists will not accept is 'judgemental relativism' (ibid.), which denies that there can be any rational grounds for preferring one discourse to another, or for distinguishing between knowledge and rhetoric. Rorty's pragmatism offers one reason why we should accept one theory rather than another: 'because it works' (1979, p. 176). The difference between Rorty and critical realists is simply that Rorty would say it is true because it works, while realists would say it works because (and to the extent that) it is true.

3   The aspect of critical realism which distinguishes it most clearly from other forms of realism is the way it distinguishes the objects the human sciences address. Objects of knowledge are neither our experiences *per se*, nor the events and actions which bring them about. These constitute two domains of reality, according to Bhaskar: the empirical and the actual. To become knowledge, the empirical has to be transformed, while the 'actual' (e.g. the recent disasters in Rwanda) tends to be too detailed and over-determined to be susceptible to the grasp of science without disaggregation. It is rather the structures which, by being themselves, in their intermeshing *produce* these phenomena, of which we can have more systematic knowledge. These include, for example, capitalist economies and the many sub-structures these involve. They also include the human mind, the human body, the political and legal system of a nation, etc. These structures can be understood in terms of their causal powers, i.e. relationally rather than directly through perceptual categories. Yet that which brings about effects must exist, and these 'objects' are *real*; for Bhaskar, paradigmatically so. 'To be is not to be perceived, but rather (in the last instance) just to be able to do' (Bhaskar, 1989, p. 12). Causal relations here are not understood in terms of empirical regularities, but in terms of expressions of the tendencies of things (including people). This means that something may have tendencies which are never realized, or only in some instances; or effects which sometimes take one form and sometimes another, depending on the counter-tendencies operating. Marx's discussion of the lowering of the rate of profit would be one example (1966, p. 211). Another would be the effect of childhood trauma on later experience. Such an understanding of causality dissolves the old free-will/determinism debate, by rejecting its positivist foundations.

The project of this book

A critical realist position makes the project of this book possible and meaningful, though ambitious. I set out to compare various theories of the workings of the human mind with reference to their social assumptions and their political implications. I do this in the belief that both social theorists and political activists need to be informed by psychological theory. If they are not using psychological assumptions openly and deliberately, they will do so covertly and unawarely. This position is spelt out and defended in Chapter 2. If, as I argue, human psychological capacities must be taken into account in any adequate social theory of agency, so must the mediating, enabling and constraining environment of language, culture and social structure be taken into account in any adequate psychological theory. My purpose, though, is not merely to bring sociological considerations to bear on the literature of psychotherapeutic theorizing, nor to use the latter to challenge academic sociology. It does include these sub-purposes, for I think the rigid conventional split between disciplines can inhibit social theory while at the same time encouraging eclecticism. More importantly, my aim is to set these theories of human nature in the political context of late-twentieth century environmental threat and to draw out their strategic and tactical implications for critical scrutiny.

In this book I side with the emancipationist position that we should actively strive to transform society, in particular the worldwide social structures that fuel the destruction of the environment. Quietism or local-only politics have unintended global consequences of a serious nature. By the same token, new social movements should not be automatically supported simply because they represent resistance to current forms of domination, but need to be assessed in terms of their aims and possibilities singly and in combination. All thinking about the world makes universal claims, all value judgement universalizes. Alas, there is no simple way to ensure that emancipatory projects do not turn into their opposites. But one thing that can, I think, reduce the danger is to theorize about psychological human nature, the structure of the mind, instead of denying its sociopolitical relevance.

Chapter 2 is organized around the three pillars of political discourse, *what is*, *what should be* and *what can be*. Under the first heading, it argues that environmental destruction poses an extreme and imminent danger to our world and to human societies. Under most ethical schemata, certainly according to any that rest on conceptions of human needs, the change to societies that are both just and sustainable should be. But is such change possible? This is discussed first in terms of structural features of capitalism and socialism, then – very briefly – in terms of human psychological capacities. Concepts of human nature have tended to be rejected, for good reason, when they present human desires, emotions and notions of rationality as invariant and ahistorical. In critical realist terms this is an empiricist conception of human nature, focusing on appearances and events rather than the structures that give rise to them. Chapter 2 argues that human nature is constituted by both psychological and social structures, each mediated through the other. At any one period their combined tendencies affect what intentional social change can and cannot be imagined, wished for and brought about. Chapter 3 focuses on the concept of health, the deep contradiction between the everyday concept of health as 'normal' functioning and concepts of positive health. The former is culturally relative, the latter universal and critical. In relation to environmental threat, the denial which allows normal functioning also acts to prevent criticism and change.

Western psychotherapeutic discourses theorize psychological structures and their relationship to social structures *via* these contradictory concepts of health. I have chosen to compare some of these theories, which all have thought-provoking things to say about the scope and limits of human agency and alternative social futures. Theories of psychotherapy are partly determined by clinical practice and bear a tangential relationship to the social sciences. They offer characterizations of psychic structures and their causal powers, but tend to be pragmatically unaware of the range of variation in social contexts within which these powers and tendencies are exercised. Yet if I am right about the interdependence of the social and the psychological, an adequate psychological theory has to be non-reductionist at the very least and to have some recognition of the varying *effects* of the causes it identifies. In other words, it has to recognize the place of the social, even if it cannot offer detailed knowledge of it.

In Chapters 4 and 5 I discuss the work of Freud, Anna Freud, Klein and other object-relations theorists, attempting to spell out their assumptions about the social environments within which their generalizations hold good. This issue is addressed in their work in terms of the relationship between the internal and the external, which is significant in any theory of agency and in any attempt to assess the possibility of radical social change. In particular, I discuss the political implications of Freudian and Kleinian notions of the unconscious meaning of environmental damage and environmental repair. Chapter 6 discusses Lacan and briefly touches on the work of some post-Lacanians. As a structuralist, Lacan attempts to specify the inner nature and causal power of his objects of study. You might expect a psychoanalyst to study people, or at least the human psyche, but Lacan attempts to undermine the power of conscious agency and simultaneously to displace the causal powers of the unconscious mind from the psyche to language. From an environmentalist point of view this returns us to postmodern pessimism.

In Chapter 7 I draw on the work of Maslow, Rogers, Perls and Berne and in particular on their critical use of the concepts of positive health and the 'true self'. If a striving for domination is arguably one unacknowledged aspect of the project of human emancipation, Frosch and others have argued that its very heart is rotten: an idealist dream of the whole harmonious self in permanent concord with society. I discuss the implications of humanistic psychology for environmentalism. Chapter 8 turns to radicals in both psychoanalytic and humanistic camps and inevitably back to the relationship between internal and external. Four sorts of radical theories are discussed, which between them address gender, racial and class oppression, all aspects of the *status quo* of environmental threat. Radicals try to describe the mechanisms of social reproduction of oppressive structures, as the effects of both social and psychic structures, mediated through each other. This approach often allows them to propose weak points which can be used in formulating strategy and tactics.

A common weakness of radical theories is a tendency to fall into a deficit model, which presents the oppressors as relatively healthy while the oppressed as permanently disempowered by oppression. I discuss radical theories which avoid this trap. Chapter 9 reviews the theories and their implicit views of the current world situation, of human capacities and social possibilities and the processes through which we could build a sustainable future. What sort of evidence do we, as non-clinicians interested in social change, need before we cast our strategies in the light of any one of these theories? And what positions have green movements actually taken? I discuss the implicit or explicit psychologies of the British Green Party, ecofeminism, social ecology and deep ecology. In conclusion, I argue for a version of the radical view, according to which a reversal to environmental destruction requires a movement which addresses both internalized and external relations of oppression simultaneously – and effectively.

Chapter 2

Starting points

Political discourse tends to start from a characterization of *what is*, to either assume or argue *what can be* and to draw on these in arguing *what should be*. This is the format I propose to follow in this chapter, in order to show that ending environmental destruction is now a component of almost all political and ethical positions and that this injunction requires us to re-examine our theories of agency. For if human beings are incapable of ending the threat to our environment, if *what should be* cannot be, then to argue that it should be becomes vacuous. To determine the extent of our power to change our own social world requires an investigation of *what is*, not only of the forms of that social world itself but also of human psychological tendencies and capacities.

What is?

Earlier societies have had apocalyptic visions that have sometimes become realities. Contemporary societies face the accelerating possibility of social death. One authoritative statement about the reality and extent of the threat to all human cultures and to the survival of the human species itself was the 1987 Brundtland report 'Our Common Future', by the World Commission on Environment and Development (WCED). Throughout, it carefully documented signs of progress and hope, with what deep ecologists have described as 'unjustifiable optimism' (Sessions, 1995, p. 411). Infant mortality is falling overall, human life expectancy is lengthening, global food production is now increasing faster than the population grows, and so on. But:

> the same processes that have produced these gains have given rise to trends that the planet and its people cannot long bear . . . in terms of absolute numbers there are more hungry people in the world than ever before . . . the gap between rich and poor nations is widening – not shrinking –

and there is little prospect, given present trends and institutional arrangements, that this process will be reversed. There are also environmental trends that threaten to radically alter the planet, that threaten the lives of many species upon it, including the human species. (WCED, 1987, p. 2)

The authors went on to describe the increasing rate of deforestation, which causes droughts and flooding; the incredibly rapid and continuing transformation of productive dryland into desert; global warming; the depletion of the ozone layer, the toxic wastes contaminating the human food chain and underground water tables 'beyond reach of cleansing'; the pollution of the very air we breathe; and the ever present threat (true even now) of nuclear disasters and nuclear war. They showed that poor people suffer most from environmental degradation and inevitably respond to it by self-defensive measures that increase it – like cutting down all available wood for fuel. On these grounds they argued (parting here with deep ecologists) that poverty is environmentally dangerous, that the human social world cannot afford it, any more than it can afford the spiralling wants of the industrialized countries. Development and growth are essential to reduce poverty, even to stop it increasing. But development will not reduce poverty unless it involves redistribution within and between countries. Any effect it does have will be only temporary in reducing poverty and may rebound to increase it in the long run, unless growth and development are 'sustainable', respecting the environment as a constraint on human possibilities. In its measured tones the Commission laid out what it considered the minimum actions:

> that must be taken to reduce risks to survival and to put future development on paths that are sustainable. Yet we are aware that such a reorientation on a continuing basis is simply beyond the reach of current decision making structures and institutional arrangements, both national and international. (WCED, 1987, p. 23)

The Brundtland report seems gloomy enough to the lay reader and the destructive trends it described have become further advanced in the intervening years.

In *The Evolutionary Dynamics of Complex Systems* C. J. Dyke offers a way of conceptualizing environmental degradation. He describes 'dissipative structures' as systems which use a background flow of matter and energy to sustain, maintain and reproduce their internal coherence. Dissipative structures include tornadoes, people, cities and economic systems. These systems maintain their internal order at the cost of increasing the disorder of their environment, since they do so by 'utilising an ambient energy flux and dissipating degraded forms of that energy to their environment' (Dyke, 1988, p. 114). Such structures need a sink for waste as well as a source of wealth or energy. They work by transforming the source into waste. When the source runs out, their structure changes – things fall apart. Recycling, conservation can only slow this process down.

What should be?

For my purposes here the exact details of *what is* do not matter. The evidence is overwhelming that, for the first time in human history, we are facing a danger to our whole species and its home. Our moral and political response depends very much on whether we believe this to be our only home and on who we conceptualize as 'we' – who we let into our moral community. If our wider home includes life after death, then the meaning of our current situation may only be discoverable later or elsewhere, or may be beyond human deciphering. In that case we may refer to revelation for a response to what now seems to be.

If our moral community includes non-human beings such as animals and plants, or even the inanimate, if we attribute inherent value to the non-human environment (as in deep ecology), a wide range of possible moral responses to environmental destruction opens out (e.g. Naess, 1995b). We may take the view that not only animals but even rivers and mountains have (either or both) rights or intrinsic value. We may believe that the preservation of existing ecosystems and/or biodiversity are as important, or more important, than human survival. In practice, though, both religious moralities and ecocentric moralities have some ground in common with anthropocentric ethics: they agree that environmental destruction *should not be*:

> their policy consequences are not necessarily different. If we are to fulfil all our obligations to future generations, anthropocentrics will have to adopt attitudes to non-human nature more characteristic of ecocentrism. If 'deep greens' are to avoid the pitfalls of misanthropy and ecological authoritar-ianism, they must accept that the moral claims of human beings are at least equal to those of the environment. (Red-Green Study Group, 1995, p. 12)

For 'human-centred' ethics can recognize the aesthetic and spiritual value to humans, or even intrinsic value in the eyes of humans, of animals, plants and non-living entities. In this weak form, 'anthropocentrism' need not be instrumental (Dobson, 1995, p. 66).

The straightforward 'strong' anthropocentric position couches arguments about *what should be* in terms of beliefs about human nature (most commonly about human needs), whether understood as species-based and universal, or culturally created and sectional. In other words, environmental destruction is a bad thing because it is bad *for humans*. It prevents their needs being met in the present (this is the case for many millions alive today), and it sacrifices the future needs of the as yet unborn to those of the privileged of the present generation. Worse, the basic physical needs of many are not met, while others meet arcane constructed needs for elaborate skin care and better roses. Clearly this position gains its coherence from the assump-tion that humans' moral community must include all other humans, including future generations, and is constantly stymied by the clear evidence that this is not the case.

This humanist position meets philosophical objections not only from ecocent-rics. There is a long-standing dispute about the nature and origin of human needs which parallels the dispute about whether human nature is inherent or culturally constructed (Soper, 1981, p. 18; Doyal and Gough, 1991, p. 36). Thus Sayers refuses to distinguish, as Doyal and Gough do, between basic needs intrinsic in human nature and developed and conditional needs. He points out that:

> Needs are the negative side of ... human powers and capacities. As our powers and capacities develop, so new needs emerge; and, in turn, the growth of new needs is the spur to the development of new powers and capacities ... In this way the development of needs ... is the essential basis for human liberation. (Sayers, 1989, p. 40)

This seems far too sweeping. Surely the very question of the *distribution* of these powers and capacities, and its effects, is central to the question of their potential for liberation.

We live in a world in which the basic needs of millions of people are not being met, so that their survival is threatened, their agency severely curtailed and they are doomed to physical and mental suffering. These people are not randomly chosen, but structurally designated. Their fate is inextricably linked with the fate of those of us who are structurally destined to 'need' cars, videos and microwaves. The WCED therefore argues (but 'argues' is too strong a word for its laconic, low-key style) that their 'need' for food cannot be met because our 'need' for dishwashers and cars is met. However, just as the epidemics charted by Engels in the 1840s refused to remain tidily within the districts of the poor, so we are all threatened by the way of life which has produced such widely divergent needs. Since not only North and South, east and west, but also past, present and future are interdependent, any rational attempt to meet present needs has to be 'sustainable'. This means, according to the Brundtland report:

> development that meets the needs of the present without compromising the ability of future generations to meet their own needs. It contains within it two key concepts:
> - The concept of 'needs', in particular the essential needs of the world's poor, to which overriding priority should be given; and
> - The idea of limitations imposed by the state of technology and social organisation on the environment's ability to meet present and future needs. (WCED, 1987, p. 43)

And for us in the rich countries, 'sustainable development requires the promotion of values that encourage consumption standards that are within the bounds of the ecologically possible and to which all can reasonably aspire' (ibid.).

Kate Soper (1981) argues that it is circular to judge a society on the basis of its record of meeting human needs. For in deciding what *are* human needs: 'we are already involved in judgements of what constitutes "life" or the "good" for human beings ... implicitly asserting some statement of the form "the survival (happiness) of human beings is a good thing"' (Soper, 1981, p. 11). Soper is certainly right to point out the moral kernel in needs' concepts, but the circularity vanishes if we take human survival to be *ceteris paribus* desirable, and human suffering *ceteris paribus* bad. These are not optional, indefensible assumptions, but basic premises of non-religious moral discourse and we need not settle the more difficult issue as to what human beings need in order to thrive and flourish. As Schell writes: 'Risk of extinction has a significance that is categorically different from, and immeasurably greater than, that of any other risk ... It represents not the defeat of some purpose but an abyss in which all human purposes would be drowned for all time' (1982, p. 95).

The *ceteris paribus* clauses here are not mere tokens. Deep ecology, we shall see, challenges at least two common assumptions here: that human needs *are* being met (arguably our psychological needs to respect nature are neglected) and that other things *are* equal in a world that puts profit for humans above the survival of many, many other species. But even on the strong anthropocentric view, if we agree that human health and human survival are fundamental human needs (as we surely must since all other human choices depend on them), it must follow that if they are under threat, social change which ends that threat should be brought about. So much for *what should be*, for the precise nature of the change to be advocated must depend on the answer to the question: *what can be?*

What can be? Structures

What should but cannot be, however tragic this incapacity, is ultimately irrelevant and uninteresting. *What can be* clearly depends on *what is*, its tendencies and capacities, its immanent as well as its instantiated nature. A crucial part of *what is* (though just how crucial is part of the question at issue) consists of social and economic structures. The Brundtland report concluded that the world must move towards sustainable development. A central question emerges as to whether the present dominant social and economic system – capitalism – is capable of doing so and, if not, whether some other sort of system could do better. There is a gap, though, between devising theoretical parameters for a system and its realization, with all the unforeseen circumstances and unintended consequences (Giddens, 1990, p. 153), a gap in which postmodernists see the looming spectre of modernity. And even if human ingenuity can devise appropriate goals, whether we are collectively capable of reaching them is a further question. For the moment, though, let us review the gloomy prospects of structures we already know.

The Brundtland report is ambiguous. On the one hand it says that the necessary minimum actions are beyond the scope of existing institutional structures, but all its suggestions depend on the reformability of these structures and the system they are part of. Major industrial countries have to change their lending policies completely so that resources can flow from rich to poor without requiring the austerity programmes that ultimately widen the gap. There must be a reduction in protectionism, compensatory financing must be used to even out economic shocks, to avoid the overproduction of non-renewable commodities, and so on (WCED, 1987, pp. 82–5), requirements which sound very like asking the leopard to change its spots (Pepper, 1993, p. xi). Can international capitalism, which has immeasurably speeded up the ecological threat, now forego short- and medium-term profitability and competition and bring about the changes required?

One possible precedent might be the Industrial Revolution in Britain, which in its early years was destroying the very labour force which made its profits. To do what was rational for the class would have been economic suicide for individual capitalists. Legislation bound all and reined in exploitation to a sustainable level. But in the absence of a world State to enforce analogous measures, the Commission is asking international capital (and national capitals and their governmental representatives) not simply to increase the costs of production by including ecological considerations, not simply to write-off existing debts and change the conditions of lending, not simply to increase aid to developing countries and to gear it to sustainable development, but to redistribute power within and between countries. The Commission does not ask whether the considerations that sway an individual in private life will also sway them when representing sectional corporate interests. It addresses the major industrial countries as if they were reasonable individuals, politely asking them to give up their destructive greed.

The enormity of this is even more striking when we consider the deep ecologist rejection of 'sustainable development' as an aim. Sessions (1995) argues that the very idea depends 'on uncritical and unexamined anthropocentric assumptions . . . [it] travels the "easy road" of political compromise that fails to deal adequately with the ecological crisis' (Sessions, 1995, p. 412). This unsustainable notion of sustainability was to dominate and divert the Rio conference, underlining the distinction between deep ecology and an environmentalism which still makes nature no more than a source of goods and services for human economic development. The North expects its present way of life to continue, while the South, in the name of social justice, demands to follow the same path. Yet in the South, development since the Brundtland report has only increased the disparity between rich and poor (Sachs, 1993). Sustainability is only meaningful if it is *ecological* sustainability, aimed at protecting the richness and diversity of life forms (Naess, 1995a). If the Brundtland report is unrealistically optimistic in relation to 'sustainable development', how much more do its proposals fall short of the requirements of 'wide ecological sustainability'?

If capitalism cannot stop destroying the world, what about socialism? Marxism used to have a glib explanation of environmental degradation. The capitalist economic system is structurally obliged to expand production, always in the service of profit, sucking the natural wealth from the world and spitting out the pips, the skeletons of fish and ships, the poison of outdated weapons supposed to protect the profit of sections of that system. Capitalism has created the material base to meet human needs, but the contradiction between the forces and the relations of production make it impossible for it to do so. Its propensity to create deserts, to make whole areas of the world its 'sink' and to make whole peoples and groups part of its consumable capital, is attributed to this contradiction. The materialism of Marxism addresses the initial conditions and the internal dynamics of that 'dissipative structure', the world economic order, but not its boundary conditions. Here is a great gap in that materialism, which accepts the capitalist idea of the infinite development of the forces of production (Benton, 1989). But as Dyke (1988) says, the sensible management of resources, which means sustainable development based on renewable energy, renewable wealth, is:

> a basic constraint on human life. This is what it means to establish a continuity between biology and society – not the reduction of social life to biology, but the recognition of the shape of the possibility space through which social life has to pass, a space with ecological determinants. (Dyke, 1988, p. 140)

On its record, the socialism of the 'command economy' – the only socialism we have experienced – cannot deliver the goods and destroys the environment in the course of attempting to do so. Tragic accounts of the effects of pollution in the ex-USSR and in Eastern Europe have now emerged. Actually existing socialism, which made the great and inspiring claim of meeting the needs of all the people, produced its own varieties of racism, women's oppression and imperialist domination, did not consistently provide either bread or roses and squandered and contaminated its people's natural treasures. As Sayers says (1990, p. 46), to refuse it the name of socialism is cold comfort. From a deep green point of view this convergence was predictable, since both systems attempt to satisfy human needs by maximizing economic growth. There is no reason to believe, as Bookchin does, that eliminating social injustice would entail accepting that there are limits to growth (Dobson, 1995, p. 170).

Deep ecologists must be, in one way or another, opposed to large-scale, industrial capitalism. However, they may see the answer in terms of small-scale capitalist enterprises, which accept limits to growth, to consumption and to population and are sufficiently small-scale and participatory to allow people actually to experience the effects of their actions. The structural argument then becomes whether small-scale capitalism is a possibility, or whether it must always lead to capital concentration and domination of the profit motive; whether forms of socialism, anarchism or other unnamed types of economy can allow us to carry on human social life without sawing off the very branch we sit on.

What can be? Human capacities

What is socially and politically possible is determined by several levels of reality: by the requirements of human physiology; by the natural environment which determines what resources are available to meet these requirements; by the culture, including the level of technological development; by social and economic structures, which establish which groups have access to technology and to environmental resources; and lastly by our psychological nature. True, our thoughts, feelings, abilities and dispositions are formed by our lives and the society we live in; but not from nothing. The ways in which we experience our situation and respond to it are not infinite. They are based in a human physical and psychological nature, which establishes the opportunities and the limitations of politics. Social and political theory has always made assumptions about human motivation and human responses: about human nature, in fact, even when (as now) to do so openly was highly unfashionable and politically incorrect.

It is understandable that poststructuralism should reject ideas of human nature along with notions of the human subject. Once you blur the distinction between discourse and practice, and between language and the world, and see the body as itself socially constructed, obviously the concept of human nature must go out of the window (Fuss, 1989, p. 3). Our embodiment is central to our subjectivity and to our agency. It is our relationship as material beings to our material environment that determines the range of human forms of life. Human physical nature is the raw material of culture. Without this common nature and comparable relationship to the natural environment, translation between languages and cultures would be impossible instead of merely difficult. It is far more surprising to find materialists denying the shared nature of members of the human species. Such an argument splits:

> humanity from the natural world – in particular from other species, which
> . . . are never denied to possess an intrinsic nature – and functions in this
> respect exactly like . . . theological conceptions . . . any genuine material-
> ism must insist that human beings, for all that is distinctive about them as
> a species, and for all of their traits, activities and relationships which can
> only be explained by specificities of society and history, are nevertheless,
> like all other species, material and natural beings; irredeemably rooted in
> a given biological constitution; absolutely continuous with the rest of the
> natural world. (Geras, 1983, p. 97)

If we recognize our biological nature, which links us with other species despite our distinctness, we must also recognize our psychological nature as the source of the social characteristics we think of as paradigmatically human. Social structures did not spring fully armed from the head of Zeus: they are the product of the interaction of beings who are inherently and necessarily social. Just as sociological explanations assume the embodiment of human agents, without spelling this out, so they also assume a common psychological nature, biologically based. This common nature is the raw material of experience, of the construction of subjectivity, the set of rules according to which the self develops in response to its social environment.

Our human nature, in both its physical and psychological aspects, represents the taken-for-granted underpinnings of social theory which are actually part of the entire causal picture. Marxism, for instance, assumes that people have physical needs which must be met if they are to survive, or to survive without suffering (Geras, 1983, p. 83; Doyal and Gough, 1991, p. 12); that they have some awareness of their needs and of how they can be met in their social context; and that they tend to act in ways they believe will meet these needs. It assumes they have beliefs, which are in some way based on experience and revised in the light of it. It makes a more grandiose assumption: that human beings are capable of identifying with a group or class so that in some circumstances they will risk their lives for the sake of the collective. (See Archibald, 1989, for the explication and evaluation of a whole social psychology he claims is implicit in Marx.) All these are psychological assumptions, though untheorized ones. Their psychological nature is obscured by their 'commonsense' nature, but they are no tautologies. (Some of the 'dated' assumptions of Marx and Engels, such as their belief that the industrial revolution went against nature by undermining the sexual division of labour, can now clearly be seen as psychological assumptions, just because we no longer believe them to be true.) They refer to real capacities and tendencies of human beings, not to invariant behaviour.

The actual functioning of human minds can always only be understood in relation to their social context – the province of social theory. But this is true precisely because the human mind is constituted in a certain way, because human beings are inherently social. The causal mechanisms at the level of the social institutions work through the minds and thence the actions of human beings. Our minds, by virtue of their structure, constitute the field of operation of these 'impersonal' forces. To use a phrase of Garfinkel's, psychology and social science constitute each others' possibility spaces (1981, p. 68). Or as Dyke puts it, 'pathways through the possible . . . are determined by a plurality of interpenetrating constraints deriving from many recognisable "levels" looping back and around each other' (1988, p. 64).

In Bhaskarian terms, causally generative mechanisms exist at all these recognizable levels, which are not reducible to the simplistic tripartite academic division between biology, psychology and sociology. Actual events, happenings and actions are the product of mechanisms at various levels working simultaneously and in combination. History – that is to say actual existing societies in process – is not an expression of the 'essence of man', nor is it governed by the serial decisions of 'great men'. But it can only take place within the possibility space determined by the real, discoverable powers and limits of human beings – including our psychological powers and limits.

Can human beings change society?

Structuralism saw the subject as a mere effect of structure, making agency illusory. Interactionism saw society as continually constructed by human interaction. More recently in the mainstream of the social sciences it has become an ordinary insight to insist that structure and agency are interdependent aspects of social reality.

Bhaskar and Giddens, in their related but distinct ways, both present society as external to individuals, yet created by them; while individuals are formed by society which they in turn reproduce or transform. Bhaskar describes this double movement in his 'transformational model of social activity' (1989, p. 36) and Giddens in his 'structuration theory' (1984, p. 170). Clearly such an approach makes sense in terms of the argument of the last section.

We do not choose the family we are born into, let alone its social position, the place and time, culture and language. But as even in our earliest actions and responses we take and make our place in that society, we simultaneously reproduce and modify the very forms that condition and allow our social participation. 'Society stands to individuals, as something that they never make, but that exists only in virtue of their activity' (Bhaskar, 1989, p. 34).

When we go to school, this is an intentional act on our part as well as on that of our parents. Our conscious intentions, whatever they are (to please our parents, to be big, to have companionship?), are unlikely to include reproducing the institutions of schooling. Yet this is one of the unintended consequences of our actions combined with those of many others. On the other hand, for us to have had any intentions in relation to schools, the institution had already to exist.

> Speech requires language; making materials; action conditions; agency resources; activity rules ... Thus if the social cannot be reduced to (and is not the product of) the individual, it is equally clear that society is a necessary condition for any intentional act at all. (Bhaskar, 1989, p. 34)

People develop within and through particular social structures, which offer them a particular range of options. These determine in what ways an individual can 'make a difference' by acting one way rather than another. This is why Giddens describes structure as both enabling and constraining, because it offers us opportunities as well as describing their finitude. To see English grammar, the education system, the economy or the rules of the road as only constraining is obvious nonsense. Social structures are not a narrow passageway, through which soft humans breathlessly squeeze, for humans cannot exist outside of society. As Giddens says: 'structure is implicated in that very "freedom of action" which is treated as a residual and unexplicated category in ... "structural sociology"' (1984, p. 174).

Despite this, Giddens has been criticized for overstressing human capacity to decide and act and understressing constraint – with all the conservative political implications of voluntarism, or that variety of existentialism that emphasizes the freedom of the prisoner (New, 1994). He has perhaps not sufficiently carefully distinguished between the sense in which structures themselves enable and constrain and the sense in which they express and reproduce asymmetrical power relations, which give people in some social positions far more options than others. In a sense – and Giddens is right to insist on the theoretical significance of this – as long as more than one option remains open to me in a given social situation, the structures which govern it can be said to enable as well as constrain me. As long as I can choose – even if the choice is between degradation and death – I remain an actor and enabled (to choose one of these unwanted options). Only if another hand on mine forces me to push the trigger am I *only* constrained. But in practice, as Giddens acknowledges, when we talk about constraint we are implicitly referring to motives we take for granted, such as the will to survive or the desire for certain material goods. Someone within an asymetrical power relation (a prisoner, a worker, a child) may well be 'unable to do anything other than conform to whatever the trends in question are, given the motives or goals which underlie their action' (Giddens, 1984, p. 178).

As Giddens recognizes, this view implies a certain dependence of social science on a notion of psychological, as well as material, human nature. Motivation, wishes, desires are not simply given either by our physical make-up or by our role in social structures. (In *Modernity and Self Identity* Giddens goes further down this road by attempting to integrate psychological and sociological theory. Unfortunately the only reason he offers for his choice of Erikson's theories is pragmatic (Giddens, 1991)). Bhaskar, too, notes in passing the need for the as yet undeveloped science of psychology (undeveloped in his opinion, that is) in order to theorize agency adequately (1989, p. 111). Both recognize that psychological structures exist which mediate and are mediated by social structures. This recognition opens the door to a particular form of social critique, in terms of the relationship between particular social forms and human psychological capacities. We shall explore these in the following chapters.

Human motivation is obviously key to deliberate social change, which neither 'structuration theory' nor Bhaskar's 'transformational model' do much to illuminate. Just to say that agents daily reproduce, modify or transform society is to beg the question of whether they can do so *intentionally*. Although people who conform to rules (usually) contribute to their maintenance, those who break them do not necessarily strike a blow for their transformation. Going to school helps to maintain schools but playing truant or becoming excluded do so too, as Durkheim long ago argued about crime. Admittedly the cumulative impact of a large number of people acting in similar ways (not the same thing as collective action), tends to result in modifications in structure; as where increase in unmarried cohabitation has led to changes in the law, so that unmarried heterosexual couples are increasingly treated as if they were married. In a small way these are structural changes, but their overall impact is probably to maintain the deeper *status quo*. Deviance can only have a transformative effect if, at the very least, it is articulated in the form of principles which challenge the legitimacy of the rules. Even then, some structures are more impervious to human agency than others. To understand how and in what conditions agents can deliberately change society, we need a theory of the structuring of structures.

Unless we can successfully theorize processes of social transformation, we shall be left with the rather unsatisfactory position that society is transformed by 'knowledgeable agents' (Giddens, 1984, p. 21), that this represents an 'achievement' (Bhaskar, 1989, p. 36) and that nevertheless these knowledgeable agents know not what they do, since they both change and reproduce society by mistake, unintentionally, as a side-effect of everyday social life.

Deliberate social change

On the face of it it seems all too likely that social change occurs independently of human political intentions. In 30 years of interrupted political activity, I have been associated with very few successes. A group I belonged to did raise money to send a landrover to ZANU, who subsequently took power in Zimbabwe. The anti-poll tax campaign, in which I was active, succeeded up to a point. But ZANU would have won without our landrover and the organized campaign against the poll tax was just the tip of the iceberg of sheer inability to pay, where the intention was to get by from day to day rather than to abolish the tax. So even on occasions like these when I and others are on the winning side, it seems as if we are more like the froth on the waves than the power of the sea.

The gap between the action and the desired end seems even more grotesquely huge in the case of individual action, such as my friend who, for ecological reasons, goes to the swimming pool by bus to avoid using her car, or another friend who removes all superfluous packaging at the supermarket checkout and leaves it there. In the face of such quixotic attempts society appears like a gargantuan, immovable object, thoroughly external to the individual. Or, in sociological language, 'the greater the time-space distanciation of social systems – the more their institutions bite into time and space – the more resistant they are to manipulation and change by any individual agent' or, indeed, by any collective one – a concept Giddens rejects (Giddens, 1984, p. 171).

Both Giddens and Bhaskar advocate change. Here, though, they begin to diverge (though according to Archer (1995) the overall differences between them are more significant than I have suggested). At first there is just a difference in emphasis. Both point out that social scientific critique can offer reasons for social change and can constitute a political intervention in its own right (Giddens, 1990, p. 304; Bhaskar, 1989, p. 63). If makers of a certain washing powder claim it is 'kind' to the environment and a pressure group shows that claim is baseless, one reason for buying the powder is removed. If we can also explain why and how the false belief is generated – because 'truth is a good' (other things being equal) – this offers a reason for changing the institutionalized practices which produced the false belief. And if widely known and accepted, the new knowledge is itself a step towards that, since enduring social practices depend on the beliefs of the actors involved. So 'explanatory critiques' can themselves be political interventions, in certain situations. However, Bhaskar stresses the need for conscious emancipatory practice aimed at structural change. Giddens, far more cautious in his political ambitions, emphasizes that human power to transform society is limited by the ubiquity of unintended consequences.

We cannot expect either Bhaskar or Giddens to specify conditions in which human beings can make history by intentionally changing the structures they live in and through, because there is no general answer to the question 'Can we change society?' But just as we can give no general *positive* answer ('Human beings can always wrest society to their purposes'), we can give no general *negative* one either ('human beings are incapable of making history, because unintended consequences necessarily subvert their purposes'). In an open system and a highly complex one at that, all actions will have unintended consequences, which will on occasion sabotage the purposes of the actor. Such sabotage is sometimes presented as increasingly inevitable (e.g. Giddens, 1990, p. 153). Human beliefs and intentions are part of the very social structures we may wish to change. This has always been true, but the increasing 'reflexivity of social knowledge' (in Giddens' phrase) means that articulated challenges to the *status quo* are rapidly heard, assessed and responded to by various interest groups. Attempting to bring about social change in this unstable situation is a bit like the game 'triangles', in which each player silently chooses two others and tries to form an equilateral triangle with them. Since everyone has their own triangular agenda, the situation is extremely unstable.

This is a dramatic analogy. It does not licence us, however, to confuse the *contingent* difficulty, (sometimes so extreme as to amount to a specific impossibility) of deliberately bringing about social change, with a *logical* impossibility. If reflexivity rendered intentional social change impossible in this strong sense, the degree and complexity of agents' knowledge of the relevant generative structures would make no difference. However, it is still the case that the more we know about the structures and mechanisms that, working in combination, result in the events and patterns of social life, the more chance we have of bringing about wanted change and of understanding those changes that do occur.

In general, social 'states of affairs' are easier to change than the structures that generate them. I was once part of a demonstration of mothers who occupied a road outside our children's school to demand a crossing at a place where children had been injured. My daughter's class was told by their exasperated conservative teacher to ignore the noise of 'the mummies being silly, which will get them nowhere'. In fact photographs appeared in the local press, letters were written, strings pulled and a crossing was provided fairly swiftly. No structural change was involved. The rules did not change, but they were applied slightly differently; for other, less formally acknowledged rules influenced their subsequent application.

At the other extreme, Mao Zedong and the Chinese Communist Party planned and executed land reform in China in the 1930s and 1940s. This constituted a structural change, by anyone's criteria, involving a massive shifting of resources, a radical change in power relations and the replacement of one set of social rules of how people in particular positions in the social system should conduct themselves with another set of rules corresponding to a different set of positions. There is plenty of documentary evidence that, despite a plethora of unintended consequences, in broad outline the change was desired, planned and carried out to produce the desired result. (The same cannot be said for the 'Great Leap Forward' and the 'Cultural Revolution'.) It seems, then, that human agents are capable both of bringing about change through institutional means and of overthrowing institutions which are an obstacle to the changes they desire.

In both these examples no one person brought about the change. The appearance of a puzzle comes from the fact that agency is necessarily singular. Individual persons have wants, individual persons act. If they were *obliged* to act in a certain way by virtue of their membership of a collectivity their agency would be called in question. So how can we reconcile the relative powerlessness of the singular human being with the singularity of agency? The 'Great Man theory of history' attempts to do so by suggesting that some individuals are really powerful. In their street cries of 'Maggie out!' even Mrs Thatcher's enemies colluded with the widespread view of her as holding immense personal power. But the puzzle is only apparent. What people can do depends on how they are positioned in social systems. Callinicos (1987, p. 86) contrasts 'structural' and 'natural' capacities (but we must remember their *effects* cannot be disaggregated).

Mrs Thatcher's structural capacity, by virtue of her post as Prime Minister, was different (and in some but not all ways greater) than it had been when she was a mere backbencher. She was not indispensable, as Major's succession demonstrated; nor all-powerful, since some courses of action were as firmly ruled out by her position as others were facilitated. But undoubtedly the decisions she took made a difference. In that sense, she did 'make history', as did Chairman Mao; while our little group of mothers only affected a few personal biographies. Yet the structural capacity of leaders depends on the collective exercise of the structural capacity of their followers, on the decisions of many others like the ordinary mothers on the street. Had millions of peasants not decided, for their own reasons, to follow the line of the Communist Party of China (C.P.C.), Mao's leadership would have been reduced to impotent posturing.

At any one time only certain sorts of changes are possible: *what can be* depends on *what is*. Social change has the old society as its raw material and can only go as far as the possibilities already immanent in that. Good, that is to say effective leaders – if we ignore for a moment the question of *what should be* – are those who make an accurate assessment of what is, *at the level of underlying structures and mechanisms, not simply phenomena*. This must include an accurate assessment of their own constituency's interests, wants and capacities. Good followers assess the adequacy of the leader's grasp of these, which may include making their own analysis. Agents can then deliberately bring about structural changes, though not just *any* such. To do so deliberately (rather than by accident) they have to have carried out an analysis of *what is* which identifies the underlying structures resulting in unsatisfactory practices and states of affairs, the immanent possibilities of the situation and strategy and tactics based on these and their own actual or potential structural capacities. Having analysed, they have to *act*, to critique, expose, persuade, lead, join, refuse or do otherwise. How effective such action is depends on the adequacy of the analysis, on the constant use of feedback and on the extent to which unforeseeable determinations occur.

Motivation and the need for psychology

Why do agents want to bring about change in the first place? Bhaskar contrasts 'interests' and 'wants', that notoriously difficult couple: 'although it is a necessary truth that people act on their wants, it is not a necessary truth that they act on their interests' (1989, p. 114). On the other hand, it must be a necessary truth that, other things being equal, people *should* act on their interests. To sustain such a disjunction there must at least sometimes be painful or restricting effects of acting on wants, rather than interests. Bhaskar describes a non-alienating society as one in which 'people self-consciously transform their social conditions of existence (the social structure) so as to maximise the possibilities for the development and spontaneous exercise of their natural (species) powers' (1989, p. 47).

It follows that oppressive structures are those which systematically prevent such an exercise of powers, *whether or not the people concerned are aware of it*. By the same token it must be in people's interests to act to end the oppressive structures that limit them.

Such a concept of 'real interests' is no more than a placeholder, with little substantive content. But by anchoring interests in human capacities it offers a subtler and potentially richer account than the reductionist economistic notion of 'interests' shared by vulgar Marxism and simpler versions of rational-choice theory. Anyone who distinguishes wants from interests then has to explain why people do not always act on their interests. Rational-choice theory has sometimes responded to the criticism that people simply do not act like *homo economicus* (i.e. instrumentally to maximize their economic interests), by reinterpreting the concept of interests in terms of 'wants' or 'desires', whatever these may be, assuming that such non-economic 'preference structures' are either idiosyncratic or acquired through socialization (Elster, 1982, p. 465). The trouble is that this retreat to the subjective puts political ambitions, secret desires and everyday culinary tastes on the same level and treats them much as if they were money: as commensurable and calculable. By trying to avoid the difficulties of an 'ontologically deep' model, it produces tautology: 'I act to get what I want . . .'

In the main people behave in complex, overdetermined, symbolic, repetitive and unexpected ways that only an 'ontologically deep' theory has a chance of explaining. Such a theory must be able to justify distinguishing interests from wants. It must be able to explain why people sometimes act against their interests and when they are likely to do so. A worked-out notion of interests would have to include the individual's needs for physical survival – basic human needs – and for a satisfying cultural life which allows, as Bhaskar says, the development and use of the person's capacities. Arguably, social participation is itself a basic need. It must also be in an individual's real interests not only to thrive herself, but for all those in her moral community to thrive.

But this is to multiply placeholders in a way far too condensed and untheorized to be satisfactory. For example, on inspection all notions of interests turn out to be complex constructions, in which economic interests are no more straightforward than others. How do we come to choose between money in our pocket or a greater social wage? Or between either of these and a safer or less-polluted future? Or between our wants for our children and the requirements of the organization we work for? Culturally accepted constructions of material or economic interests play a major role in *rationalizations*, since in many cases these are socially accepted as good, or at least intelligible, reasons for acting. But if we try to explain support for Conservative transport policy, for instance, which has vastly increased the number of cars in the UK, we will probably find that while some of its supporters will accrue considerable material benefits, many will not. Even those who will benefit economically stand to lose in other ways that might be expected to have motivating value. They may have or expect to have grandchildren whom they love, whose lives are likely to be deleteriously affected by increased pollution. The processes through which people select and avoid information to construct their subjective interests cannot be modelled in terms of weights and balances. People's ideas of their interests may well be influenced by inappropriate, ancient fears (of feeling humiliated again, of losing parents' love or social approval) as well as appropriate ones (of contributing to the undesired outcomes of environmental destruction and eventual social death).

The conclusion of this chapter is that in order to answer *political* questions about what is and what should be, we need to theorize psychological human nature. To sum up: to explain – or to bring about – deliberate social change we need to know a lot about *what is*. This crucially includes human motivation: what makes humans want to bring about one state of affairs rather than another. This is a complex matter which necessitates distinguishing *wants* from the evaluative concept of *interests* and going further by asserting both that interests are mediated by social context *and* that people can be mistaken about their own interests. Such a move can only be justified in terms of a conception of what human beings are like, of what they need in order to thrive, with implications for *what should be*. All this requires more than a vague philosophical anthropology: it requires *psychological* theorizing.

Revolutionaries, reformers and political activists generally, whatever their standpoint, have always been interested in psychology in a pragmatic, eclectic way. So have advertisers, often with striking effect, although they would arguably rather manipulate rationalizations than replace them with good reasons. Isn't a casual, eclectic psychologizing enough? No. If we want to minimize the unintended consequences of our political action, we surely need to take all findings of the human sciences seriously – and discriminatingly. Sociological theory, too, takes psychological knowledge for granted in its assumptions about agency, usually without admitting it is doing so. This failure to specify *which* psychological theory is being assumed inevitably obscures the way psychological structures and mechanisms enter into the determination of *what is* and *what can be*. What these psychological structures are, then, is vitally important to the questions of whether we *can* change social structures and whether we can sustain the changes we make.

Which psychological theories? Many sorts of psychology contribute to our knowledge of what human beings are like. The most relevant here are those that address the formation of subjectivity and human tendencies and capacities as *moral agents*, rather than as perceivers, learners and rememberers. Of these I have chosen to focus on theories of psychotherapy, which originate in clinical practice and are thus dedicated to the person as agent. A schematic concept of psychological health is implicit in the conclusions of this chapter. It is closely linked to the idea of freedom and self-emancipation. Bhaskar describes a free agent as one who is:

capable of realising his or her real interests (which means knowing, acting
on and bringing about a state of affairs satisfying them) (1989, p. 114)

so as to substitute 'wanted and needed sources of determination' for 'unwanted and
unneeded' ones (Bhaskar, 1986, p. 171). To be in this state of 'freedom' we have
to be 'in gear' with the causal order of the world (with *what is*), understanding
ourselves and our environment and their 'necessary tendencies'. Collier shows that
this notion of freedom is related to some psychotherapeutic conceptions of mental
health (1994, p. 193), as when someone becomes free of a disabling obsession and
is thus able to act more powerfully in the world.

The relationship is even closer. If freedom involves the capacity to realize
one's own interests and to recognize necessity, psychological health might be seen
as a necessary but not a sufficient condition for freedom, as a state in which someone knows their own interests and acts to further them, *to the extent their situation
allows,* recognizes the 'necessary tendency' of things *to the extent the available
evidence permits.* In other words, there may be external obstacles to their realizing
their own interests, but they are not sabotaging themselves. In the next chapter I
explore the relationship between health and agency and the contradictions within
concepts of psychological health.

Chapter 3

Conflicting concepts of health

Agency, health and human capacities

Human embodiment is central to our ideas of agency and so is mind: intelligence and a capacity for symbolic communication. The body is the locus of personhood, the site of the subject; it is the body that gives a point of view, however temporary, that is the medium of experience, the centre of memory and personal identity, the determinant of the possibilities of action. Whenever sociological theories talk about agents they tend to assume 'normal' bodily capacities and 'normal', i.e. healthy, functioning. Sociological writings do not bother to explain that human beings are normally bipedal and have to eat; after all, they are not written for Martians. People's physical capacities (in a particular situation, with particular technological resources) are always part of the causal preconditions of social events or processes, but this is a part that we usually bracket.

Just as importantly, *mind* is central to agency. The psychological level emerges out of the physiological, in that for their very possibility mental processes depend on certain conditions of the brain and other parts of the body. Nevertheless, because they have their own causal power and because they are affected by happenings outside the person, mental processes are distinct from the brain processes that both permit and reflect them. Neurological reductionists ignore this point:

> since all behaviour is a reflection of the patterns of activity in the brain, and this holds equally for normal, psychiatric and neurological populations, it follows that variations in behavioural patterns are manifestations of the state of equilibrium in the brain. (Gur, Levy and Gur, 1977, p. 20)

But if I panic when my mother goes into hospital, this behaviour is the result of experience, of the *meaning* of this event in my life. My brain, if we assume its functioning to be altered, is affected by my mind. The very concept of action implies that what agents do is *caused* by their internal mental states. Just as explanations of action assume 'normal' bodily capacities and functioning unless otherwise stated, they also assume 'normal' psychological capacities and functioning. Mind and body are inseparable, interdependent but irreducible to each other, and the concept of a person includes their unity in agency.

All societies have some concept of health to characterize 'the state in which individuals can be and are fully human' (Wright, 1982, p. 19) – that is, capable of doing whatever that society sees as the activities that define an accountable person of the relevant sort. If health is your state when you can do what you should do, illness is one way of characterizing the state when you *cannot*, but because this incapacity is both temporary and involuntary, you still count as a full member of society. The 'cannot' here need not have the organic aetiological overtones of the Western distinction between health and ill-health. In some societies a state of optimal functioning and capacity would be thought of as one in which no one was successfully aiming magic at you.

What counts as a practice definitional of humanness is socially constructed. In some respects such activities and states will be constructed in the same way, because of the very basic similarity of all human societies. To be a full member of *any* human society you have to be able to communicate, for example, and to be able to pay enough effective attention to the environment to get your needs met, though there are mindbogglingly various ways of doing this. But in one society you need to be able to read and in another to decipher the bush. We can imagine a world in which those without X-ray vision were disabled and those whose X-ray vision was temporarily not functioning were ill. 'Out of anthropocentric self-interest, we have chosen to consider as "illnesses" or "diseases" those natural circumstances which precipitate . . . death (or the failure to function according to certain values)' (Sedgewick, 1982, p. 30). What these values are is a cultural question, but also a question of power in a more specific sense. Cultures are not homogenous givens but processes, in which differently structurally positioned groups interpret, reinterpret, appropriate or challenge existing understandings, practices and standards. Such standards will be age- and sex-related and relative to social position. There will be some social positions which institutionalize deviance (e.g. blind musicians). Individuals will find their own levels within the culturally imposed normal range, so that a sort of normal functioning – and thus health – is possible too for the 'disabled' (Siegler and Osmond, 1976, p. 37).

'Health' in this everyday, commonest sense means 'not-illness', or the near-synonymous capacity to function normally. When someone other than a doctor asks 'How are you?' this interchange is rarely a request for information, as anyone can find out by trying the effect of giving some. People who care about us may be interested in our infected finger but most people await the ritual word – 'Fine!' – as confirmation that we are willing to take responsibility for our actions. You may not be feeling at all fine. Your back may be aching, but it often does. One of your eyes is aching too – perhaps your lenses are dirty. The same eye is twitching nearly invisibly, but irritatingly, suggesting a future of involuntary spasms. You feel hungry, which is probably more connected to what is about to be asked of you than to how much you ate at your last, not too distant meal. You are lacking in positive health, but not actually ill. 'Fine' refers to your whole embodied being: we can count on you not to faint or burst into tears; you are neither incapacitated by misery nor by 'flu.

The coming of aetiology and the mind/body split

Since the psychotherapeutic theories we will be looking at in the following chapters present their theories of psychological human nature and of the scope of agency in terms of the discourse of health and illness, I want to make a detour here to consider the question of whether, and in what sense, 'mental illness' is real. So far illness has been described as a temporary inability to take one's full part in social life. Such episodes must occur in all societies, whether they are believed to be caused by spirits, germs or an imbalance of yin and yang. They may indeed have more than one concept of involuntary social incapacity and 'illness' may be contrasted with something else, such as 'madness'. Each culture's theories will affect who is thought of as ill, who thinks of themselves as ill and even, such is the power of meaning, who becomes ill. It is only when we place our causal cards on the table that it becomes clear that the distinction between mind and body is crucial to some theories and absent in others (Foucault, 1967, p. 178; Bakal, 1979, p. 15).

The paradigm of illness in Western culture has increasingly become externally caused disease or organic malfunction. This, and only this, provides the perfect alibi for temporary breakdown of functioning. The sick role, as a concept and as an institution, reflects the hegemony of this model. The physical has become the province of medicine. The breakdown of the body is considered involuntary and exculpating even when the person was known to themselves and others to be behaving in ways likely to bring about such breakdown, such as smoking, drinking, living in cities and eating a high-fat, low-fibre diet. This intensification of the mind-body split is paradoxically accompanied by increasing acknowledgment of their unity. But the mechanical image of the body, controlled by the ghost in the machine, is powerful. It renders 'mental illness' a problematic as well as a recent category, since it seems to involve the breakdown or distortion of the ghost itself, of intentionality and thus of moral responsibility.

If Alice wants to look after her new baby, but cannot because a severe breast abscess has given her a raging temperature, there is no blemish on her moral fibre. But if there is no physical impediment, yet she neglects the little one, how are we to distinguish between 'I can't' and 'I won't'? If someone says words which make no sense and the doctor says there is nothing wrong with their brain, their mouth and tongue, then surely they could have said other, more sensible words? If someone sits in a defeated posture, hour after hour, gazing at the floor, surely they could get up, wash their face and get on with life? These questions, this irritation, are the product of a medical model of illness in which mind/body dualism is a central strand. Psychiatry is the unsteady bridge between such a model and opposed aetiological theories such as those of psychoanalysis.

Its compromise involves anatomizing the mind functionally, on an analogy with organs of the body, and diagnosing mental illness in terms of the breakdown of one or more dimensions of functioning (Clare, 1976, p. 19). Psychoanalysis responded to the breakdown of intentionality by radically extending the notion, so that unconscious intentions could explain behaviour (such as the neglect of a child) in opposition to conscious intentions. But psychoanalysis too fails fully to exculpate. The more effectively it renders unintelligible behaviour intelligible, breaking down the wall between the mad and the reasonable, the more our conceptions of moral responsibility and agency themselves expand to the point where we take responsibility for our unconscious wishes. For here too we are in the grip of the Cartesian split. If the cause of illness is physical, it is somehow external to the real us. If it is mental, it is ours.

The classification of illness into physical or mental illness is not phenomenologically straightforward. The names of illnesses instruct us to treat some of their aspects as essential, others as marginal: thus constipation, stooping posture and lack of energy are mere effects of depression, which is an affective disorder, while irritability, isolation and confusion are the side-effects of deafness, which is 'really' organic. Such instructions are derived from the causal theory for which the diagnostic label stands in. A modern nosology which included 'interactionist' theories might look something like this:

Table 3.1 Dualism in illness assignment

Main type of cause	Main form of illness: Physical	Main form of illness: Mental
Physical	1 Diabetes, TB, fracture, phlebitis, measles, sinusitis, deafness	3 Syphilis (GPI), brain tumour, Tourette's, Altzheimer's
Mental	2 Ulcers, hysteria, migraine, asthma, psoriasis, colitis	4 Depression, paranoia, phobias, obsessional neurosis

This tentative placing shows just how hard it is to assign illnesses, even with the long tradition of Western dualism to refer to. TB and measles cannot be accounted for in terms of pathogens alone, since far more people are exposed than become ill. The immune system, prime candidate for explaining the difference, is probably affected by our states of mind. Michael Balint describes the process of negotiation between patient and general practitioner, in which patients who have a psycholo-
~~~~ need to be ill offer various complaints until one is accepted as justifying the
tween doctor and patient – an analysis which nicely muddies the
veen boxes 1 and 4 (Balint, 1964, p. 189). Asthma and everything
ly have physical causes as well as mental ones. Cancer could go in

boxes 1 and 2; so could coronaries. Depression and anxiety could go in boxes 3 and even 1 as well as 4.

Despite the overlap of conditions, the models of causation typically invoked are different for each box. In box 1, we have a simple – and inadequate – Humean model. In box 2 (except for hysteria, which in this respect belongs in box 4), *stress* is brought in as a mediating factor between 'physiological predisposition', 'appropriate psycho-social stimuli' and disease onset (Bakal, 1979, p. 74). The resulting symptoms are not related to the original stressful experiences at the level of meaning, as Freud found hysterical symptoms to be: an ulcer results from over-acidity resulting from stress, it has no *meaning* on this psychosomatic model. What's special about box 4 is not that the conditions in it involve emotions and thinking – so do those in boxes 2 and 3. It is that the feelings, thoughts and actions of those in box 4 are seen as both intelligible and unintelligible. They are unintelligible in that they do not make sense, they are not how a 'normal' person would react: hence the diagnosis of illness. They are intelligible in that they are comprehensible as reactions to experience, sometimes referring to it in a disguised or symbolic way. A hermeneutic practice is appropriate which would be quite out of place in trying to explain, say, fear of water in rabies. That fear is not related to experience, but belongs in box 3 in which abnormal brain states affect mental functioning. In contrast, agoraphobia in women (for those who believe in box 4 at all) is convincingly related to the experience of being a woman and a housewife.

Box 4 does not oblige us to embrace psychiatric diagnostic categories, nor to accept the label 'mentally ill', but it recognizes that we can be severely disabled by experience alone, without there being anything 'wrong' with our brains or with the emergent minds that generated the rigid responses. Box 4 leaves room for theories which move from the general and individual characteristics of mind to *social* criticism. So does Box 2. Both suggest that experience and thus the social environment is implicated in psychological distress. But Box 4 allows us to go beyond deficit models most used in Box 2, where distress and disorder are caused by stress resulting from traumatic life events and unmet needs, to more complex models in which the *meaning* of what happens to us has causal salience. In such models the social environment affects what happens to people, which may be conducive or inimical to psychological health in general terms. It also provides them with the concepts to make sense of these happenings; the adequacy of these also has a crucial effect on psychological health.

Sociological theories of mental illness are often willing to treat organic illness as paradigmatic and as real, and in contrast to refuse to distinguish between 'mental illness' and intentional, willed deviance (Szasz, 1976). Labelling theory suggests that the diagnosis of 'mental illness' usually takes some 'residual misconduct' as a starting point, i.e. behaviour which is considered unintelligible by those doing the labelling. This may be because of the ignorance, ethnocentrism or lack of imagination of the labeller, but once the label is given, it has its own power to affect the person and those around them (Smith, 1978; Millett, 1991, *passim*). Articles in the 1970s used to stress that the powerful (or simply the lucky) were free to be eccentric but the powerless might find themselves labelled 'mad' and incarcerated

(Grey, 1967). Medical anthropologists have argued that standards of normality were culture-bound and that criteria of intelligibility are internal to discourse (Marsella and White, 1982, p. 3; Coulter, 1973, p. 149). Feminists have shown that diagnoses of 'mental illness' have long been part of the everyday armoury of sexism (Chesler, 1972; Showalter, 1987, p. 5). All this has been powerfully demonstrated in general terms, yet I want to insist on the *reality* of the states and experiences that are often clumsily bundled into the categories of box 4.

The concept of 'mental illness' is indeed used to justify many oppressive practices and to frighten the not-yet-stigmatized into conformity. But in rejecting the label of illness, critics often refuse any specificity to the states that are so labelled. *Standards* of health are socially constructed, but the episodes our society terms 'illness' often (but not always) have a reality beyond their social attribution. It is because people do become unable to carry on that all societies have some such concept.

States of psychological distress or rigidity are real and often prevent people functioning in the society which played a major part in their production. Sometimes they are transient and disappear when the situation which evoked them passes. Sometimes they result in a relatively enduring set of ways of responding which (usually with help from outside) keep the person trapped in a distressing situation. What are they? They are states in which we cannot use all our capacities to think, feel and create, but are channelled into rigid responses and unrealistic ways of seeing, explicable only in terms of past events and the present desire to avoid emotional pain. These states may themselves bring about (a different sort of) pain, or may be experienced as comfortable and safe. From a critical realist point of view, the key point is that they are severely limiting.

Such states are commonplace, sometimes even permanent, among non-labelled individuals. However, some of them cannot be reconciled with local conceptions of normal functioning. To that extent the idea of 'illness' has a certain legitimacy, but has to be rejected on two grounds. First, it is coloured with assumptions of organic aetiology or moral inadequacy and the oppressive use of the medical model. Second, it covers up the fact that such states are just as common, though their form will differ, among the labellers as the labelled. For these reasons I shall not use the term 'illness' when I speak in my own voice (but I shall in exposition of psychoanalytic theorists). Instead I shall speak of 'psychological distress' and 'psychological health', in full recognition that these categories are not given but disputed. I recognize that psychiatric taxonomy plays its own role in the creation and the duration of the conditions it names. It is still the case that Box 4 type states, which prohibit normal functioning, are real states of the individual and that there are limits to relativism in determining what counts as psychological health.

The bio-medical model has rightly been criticized for seeing health as an individual matter (Wright, 1982, p. 52) and for seeing the individual only:

> as monad, a container holding the mechanisms of personality within itself and surounded by an environment consisting of other monads. Accordingly, disease is something going on within a person; it is to be looked for in

the malfunctioning of the 'parts' of his personality and not in the entire relationship between self and the world. (Kovel, 1981, p. 86)

Nevertheless health and ill-health *can* validly be described as states of the individual – not in contradistinction to the relationship between self and the world, but as one aspect of it. Certainly individuals are not monads and society is internal to them as well as part of their environment. Nor can episodes of inability to function be understood, let alone treated, without looking at the relationships between the person and her social world. But the person in question is in a real state of mind, which may be normatively described, in different cultural contexts, as healthy or unhealthy. However described, it is real and causally generative: it determines what she currently can and will do. To deny this is to abolish the subject and the causal efficacy of agency. The fact that psychologically disabling states are located within the individual is perfectly consistent with their *causes* being social and with discrimination being part of the official process of assessment. Thus sexism may play a role both in the production of psychological distress and in how it is categorized and treated (Busfield, 1989).

Mental health and 'illness': The limits of relativism

Conceptions of mental as of physical health vary between societies, cultures and individuals. But just as there are some bodily conditions that no conceivable society could consider healthy, because they are incompatible even with the most specialized or minimal form of agency, so there are psychological states which prohibit *any sort* of normal functioning, in Timbuctoo or Tokyo, until they are addressed (Opler, 1969, p. 98). Human beings share forms of life rooted in our common nature, in the sorts of creatures we are and the basic needs we share. By virtue of this communality we are potentially intelligible to each other; and these common forms of life allow translation and understanding between cultures, even though something – we can never know how much – is lost in translation. If to be bodily healthy your heart must beat, your lungs and all your vital organs work to sustain your life, to be psychologically healthy you must at least be able to participate actively, intelligibly and accountably in the society in which you live, even if your participation takes the form of fierce and active rejection. You must share with at least some others at least some beliefs about how things are and how things should be. More important than the actual beliefs is agreement with others about how knowledge is reached, a shared epistemology and the ability to *communicate* agreement or disagreement with other human beings.

If Rose paints anti-poll tax slogans on walls under cover of darkness, risking arrest, you do not have to share her political views to understand her behaviour, whether you see it as admirable or as deplorable. If she starts painting nursery rhymes on walls in broad daylight, if she tells us that the best way to achieve socialism is to jump up and down, no imaginative leap provides us with a discourse within which this makes sense. At least in some sort of schematic form, ideas of instrumental rationality – effective ways of meeting goals – are necessarily part of every cultural repertoire, even if alongside other principles and excluded from some spheres. Necessarily, because human survival depends on these sort of judgements. It is not that human beings always or even usually act in end-gaining ways. Each culture will have its own ideas of when such behaviour is appropriate and a range of acceptable reasons for behaving in other ways. In ours, 'mental illness' is rolled out when other explanations fail. Rose may behave oddly as a (risky) joke, to shock the bourgeoisie, for a bet, in a perverse mood. The point is that a reason is called for and the more often she behaves in hard-to-understand ways the more urgently we need one. To be 'well' it is not enough for Rose to habitually take action which others can recognize as goal-directed, even if inept. Her goals themselves, including the emotions which move her, have to be recognizable as human and intelligible:

> Can we categorise . . . the case of the person who says she *just* wants a saucer of mud? . . . not under the false impression that it is nutritious, nor as an aesthetic whim, nor because it is pleasant to look at or muck about in. She just wants it. (De Sousa, 1987, p. 176)

Now the question of whether behaviour, feelings, goals and judgement of reality are accurate, appropriate and intelligible is a political one and therefore highly contentious, as feminists and ex-mental patients among others have argued. The psychotherapeutic hermeneutic project is to show that the unintelligible *does* make a certain sort of sense, to explain the choice of an 'inappropriate' reaction. The radical response is often to argue that the reaction (such as post-natal depression) was, after all, appropriate. If what is appropriate is contentious, it is also a matter of degree. Someone may be unable to function for minutes, hours or days, but may not incur a diagnosis which would start them on a 'career' as a mental patient, with its own compelling logic (Goffman, 1968, p. 125). It is to some extent a question of time and place. Mild obsessionality fits some societies and some social positions; sadism and masochism can find acceptable social niches. Nevertheless people *do* experience states where they feel and act in ways no one, anywhere, would be likely to consider appropriate. Whether such states of mind are usefully described as 'mental illness' is a political as well as a theoretical question. Causal theories which explain the breakdown of functioning also offer explanations of healthy states and states in-between. Drawing a line is fraught with consequences, but the constructed nature of such divisions must not be allowed to obscure the reality and causal power of the states of mind at issue.

So far I have argued that what Western societies term 'mental illness' is socially constructed, but on the basis of real states of mind. It is not entirely culturally relative, for all societies have some common features which result in some states of mind being deviant and disabling, even if not always described in terms of illness.

This is as far as we can go on the basis of the everyday notion of health as the capacity to function normally and illness as a breakdown in normal functioning.

Normal functioning is obviously relative to social structure and culture. Each culture will ethnocentrically see its own 'normal functioning' as a universal index of psychological health. If we want to say that health is culturally relative, we have to accept each definition *for its social context* while rejecting its universalizing claim. Such crosscultural relativism has drawbacks. It will not allow us to use notions of health as a springboard for social criticism. From a relativist point of view, to describe a society as 'sick' on the grounds that it encourages or causes psychological ill-health is simply a term of abuse from the standpoint of another moral discourse. From a realist point of view, though, there may be objective cross-culturally valid criteria for mental health.

In all societies intelligent action requires a conceptual grasp of reality – knowledge. We can therefore argue that any enduring rigidities which are obstacles to the acquiring of knowledge of the environment are inimical to psychological health. Now in some societies (arguably in all) some such rigidities are culturally privileged and even institutionalized. Racism and anti-Semitism are obvious examples. People who honestly believe, despite evidence to the contrary that they would accept as such in other, less emotionally charged matters, that black people or Jews are the cause of various social problems or disasters, may function normally or well as members of the hegemonic ethnic group. While relativism obliges us to see them as psychologically healthy, critical realism does not. It enables us to go beyond the idea of health as mere normal functioning, to the idea of positive health.

Positive health versus health as normal functioning

Of course, the entire effort is to put myself
Outside the ordinary range
Of what are called statistics. A hundred are killed
In the outer suburbs. Well, well, I carry on.
. . . Still, there are many
To whom my death would only be a name,
One figure in a column. The essential is
That all the 'I's should remain separate,
Propped up under flowers, and no one suffer
for his neighbour.
                    Spender, *Thoughts during an air raid*

The World Health Organisation's famous definition of health as 'complete physical, mental and social well being' gestures at the radical possibilities of a transcendental, positive concept of health, exasperating sociologists who want concepts they can use (Stacey, 1976, p. 3). Positive health is clearly distinct from the capacity to function

37

in some legitimate social niche. The notion of health as a state of full agency and capacity embraces a key contradiction: that between health as normal functioning and positive health.

Oliver Sacks (1982) describes profoundly ill, often stuporous patients suffering from post-encephalitic syndromes, for whom the 'wonder drug' L-DOPA led to a sort of 'awakening', often to a wonderful sense of full health, followed by difficulties that were sometimes so severe that the patient asked for the drug to be stopped. After L-DOPA:

> the patient ceases to feel the presence of illness and the absence of the world, and comes to feel the absence of his illness and the full presence of the world . . . the awakened patient turns to the world, no longer occupied and pre-occupied by his sickness . . . the world becomes wonderfully vivid again. (Sacks, 1982, pp. 214–15)

Health at first seemed to be a thing in itself, miraculously restored to these patients, but on reflection appears as a state in which a person is thoroughly in the world, focused outward on to present reality, aware of her body but not preoccupied with it, remembering the past but not continuing to live in it. To put it another way, positive health is the state in which disease and distress are not limiting our being in the world, in which we can use all our potential. But which potential? Our potential to hurt and maim other people, perhaps? Since anything human beings can do can be regarded as their potential, and since not all such potential can be fulfilled simultaneously, such a concept of positive health depends on a model of psychological human nature and wellbeing and of the relationship between human capacities. While health-as-normal-functioning is largely culturally relative in content, concepts of positive health thus point towards human capacities as transsocial and variously realized in particular societies and social situations. They can therefore have enormous critical force.

The internal states of any individual are inextricably linked with the social environment. Health is a state of the individual, but it is never *only* individual: normal functioning is relative to social organization, crucially including the organization of production (Leonard, 1984, p. 86) and the prevailing power relationships which define the 'normal'. Our opportunities to develop and use our capacities, our ideas of wellbeing and the possibilities of realizing them, depend on these prevailing forms of social organization. It is not then the case that normal functioning involves a certain amount of health, say x, and positive health a much greater amount, say x + y. Normal functioning frequently militates *against* positive health, as radicals have often argued (Laing, 1961, p. 23). It may represent not only a capacity, but also an incapacity – to act otherwise, to break the rules, to criticize and rebel; extensions of moral responsibility. It is precisely the demands of 'business as usual' that stifle our vision of our needs and the means to their achievement.

Chapter 2 reviewed the ecological argument that current trends will lead to environmental disaster. The first psychological requirement of structural change to environmental destruction is awareness: that we see what is happening. But now we encounter an interesting fact: denial. Changes in communication systems have vastly increased the number of people who know about environmental threat and whose anxiety is not alleviated by the complacency of the green consumer industry. Yet in embracing 'business as usual' (Giddens, 1990, p. 147) and applauding the goal of economic growth we are effectively denying the scale of the danger. If the threat were to an individual household, we would consider such a 'show must go on' approach quite crazy. Schell (1982, p. 4) describes:

> this peculiar failure of response, in which hundreds of millions of people acknowledge the presence of an immediate unremitting threat to their existence and to the existence of the world they live in, but do nothing about it – a failure in which both self-interest and fellow feeing seem to have died.

In *Living with the Bomb* psychotherapist Dorothy Rowe explores this process: how fears about nuclear war are usually denied, along with other painful memories and fears, in a costly process that 'pushes us further and further away from reality, both our external and internal reality' (Rowe, 1985, p. 46).

It might be perfectly sensible to carry on as usual if there is nothing you can do to avert a possible, but not an inevitable catastrophe. This position is suspicious because so few people ever carry out any sort of assessment of the situation and of their own power to change it: the denial does not even let them contemplate the situation sufficiently to assess it. The mechanisms are familiar: we turn away from information that depresses us, that might terrify us were we not effectively numbed by the diurnal round of business as usual. Normal functioning thus *requires* denial on a massive and limiting scale. In Chapter 2 I posed the question 'What can be?' It is certain that effective halting of current trends requires a clear awareness of *what is* and a focus on *what should be*. Yet the entire agenda of national elections, the stated aims of the supposedly opposite parties, ignore the unsustainable nature of business as usual.

But *is* this so crazy? What about people knowingly facing imminent but un-avoidable death and consciously deciding to carry on as usual? However, denial is not at all the same thing as 'continuing as usual' because on careful investigation you cannot do anything to prolong life and the way you live is already the best way. Denial magically tries to restore the *status quo ante* by forbidding any serious con-sideration of the feared possibility. We plan for our children's transition to adult-hood, ignoring the fact that they may face devastating changes, these children of the microwave and the video, for which they are as unprepared as we. Some of us look forward to our grandchildren while we continue to behave in ways which threaten those future citizens' very existence. As can happen in the face of individual death, feelings of powerlessness in relation to the threat to our collective survival trigger denial, which robs us of the information we need to use our actual power. But while as individuals we are not allowed to deny our age – compulsory retirement, senior citizens' concessions and the general dismissal of the old making it extraordinarily difficult – in the case of the threat of social death, denial is institutionalized. To suggest its relevance to our thinking about our children's education or our change of car is as intrusive and in as bad taste as parading a skeleton at the dinner table. On the one hand our widespread denial is incompatible with positive psychological health, in that it forces us into desperate, distorted and ultimately mad positions. But on the other hand it feels crazy to question the very premises of our lives and all our institutions, which are that the quest for growth must go on indefinitely and that the present international economic order is an unchangeable fact of life. Denial *is* normal functioning.

A contrasting model of rational behaviour is offered by many mothers of very sick children who have made themselves experts on the child's illness, have refused to accept the limits imposed by the actual state of resources and current diagnosis and treatment, have investigated alternatives, fundraised for better equipment or for travel to another country where better treatment was available, have set up associations and support groups – have used their power to the full to save their children and other people's children. The equivalent response to the social threat would necessarily involve collective political action, an area where many people feel especially and completely powerless. The fear of being thought crazy and of actually being crazy; the fear of opposing authority; the fear of thinking about the unthinkable combine to hold us passive.

We come up against the double and contradictory nature of 'mental health'. If we simply mean by the term adjustment to the society you live in and the absence of debilitating illness, then denial plays an important role in our everyday preservation of sanity. If we mean more, if we take psychological health to involve facing reality and acting effectively to bring about survival and a life worth living, denial is incompatible with it.

Freud, as we shall see, took the ability to face reality as a key criterion of mental health. In an early work he pointed out the difficulty of thinking about unpleasant and painful things. Like other creatures, we want to avoid pain. The development of consciousness and language (and now of mass communications) gives us extra dimensions in which to feel it. In *The Interpretation of Dreams* Freud described the thinking of the unconscious mind (the 'primary process') as governed by the pleasure principle, aiming at the real or hallucinated fulfilment of instinctual wishes. Our conscious thinking (the 'secondary process') is also affected by the pleasure principle, but it aims at the satisfaction of wishes in real life, even if they have to be modified to make that possible (a constant flow of cups of tea replacing milk and nipple). For this real satisfaction to be achieved – which is essential if we are to survive and thrive – our conscious thinking has to be able to distinguish between the real and the imaginary. According to Freud feelings, whether negative or positive, interfere with the realistic thinking process. For this reason we only allow memories to reach consciousness with a pale shadow of their original emotional charge. But this pale shadow must be allowed, for it provides information about the nature of the memory. 'The inhibition of unpleasure need not, however, be a complete one: a beginning of it must be allowed, since that is what informs the second system of the nature of the memory concerned' (Freud, 1953a, p. 601). Because thinking 'must concern itself with the connecting paths between ideas, without being led astray by the intensities of those ideas . . .' it must aim at 're-stricting the development of affect in thought-activity to the minimum required to act as a signal' (ibid., p. 602).

These passages will certainly not do as a complete account of thinking (some people compulsively focus on unpleasant thoughts) and this first version of the theory of repression was to be considerably revised. But they do shed light on the 'sanitizing' language of the Gulf War or of nuclear strategists. The mechanism Freud describes is comparable to Mary Daly's account of the distancing mechanism of academic scholarship (Daly, 1979, p. 133). But while Freud saw emotion as the enemy of clear thought, Daly argues (with many ecofeminists) that the supposed split between facts and values dangerously distorts reality. In politics the terms 'realism' and 'moderation' are used for beliefs which deny key aspects of modern reality and risk social death, while the words 'Utopian' and 'extreme' are used for views aimed at species survival (Schell, 1982, p. 171). Our entire culture regards the ability to separate thinking from feeling as a sign of maturity and mental health, a sign of the triumph of logic and rationality in which children and women typic-ally fall short. Every day we watch or read about representations of real horrors, without any interruption in our daily concerns, yet we are inarticulate about our long-term goals and about why 'business as usual' seems the highest good (Hoggett, 1992, p. 95). Just as on any understanding of human needs, we *need* social change to avert the danger of ecological disaster, so on any understanding of positive health, normal functioning, 'business as usual', is incompatible with it.

Is such forgetting, such denial, an unavoidable part of human nature, a short-sighted attempt at self-preservation by avoiding pain, or is it a reversible effect of our social experience? The philosopher De Sousa takes the pessimistic former view. He notes that the intensity of our desires seems to follow some sort of inverse-proportional rule. 'Other things being equal, the more distant the object – in space as well as time – the less we care' (1987, p. 225). He suggests that the biological function of emotions is to help us select between possible memories and percep-tions. If we operated like a computer-programmed robot, always choosing rational means to attain built-in goals, the amount of information we should have to scan and the number of possible choices would be endless. Emotions act as tie-breakers in decision-making. They are 'species of determinate patterns of salience among objects of attention, lines of enquiry and inferential strategies' (De Sousa, 1987, pp. 195–6). De Sousa argues that the biological function of tie-breaking can only be fulfilled by spatial and temporal 'discounting':

> If we cared about every child's death, were indignant at every govern-ment's iniquities . . . the emotional demands on us would as surely kill us as the surfeit of information would paralyse us, were it not for the fact that our organism allows only some of it to be salient at any one time. (1987, p. 232)

If De Sousa is right, our new, worldsize society has overtaken our evolutionary possibilities. We cannot develop the feeling and thinking we need to face reality and make the decisions that can ensure ourselves a future. Luckily for us there is no reason to believe he is right. We can care about long-ago massacres and injustices (as many people in Scotland and Ireland exemplify). We can cry for the deaths of faraway people. Even the denial I have been describing is far from absolute.

Conclusion

Ideas of positive health incorporate values which go beyond normal function-ing, furnishing a basis for social criticism. That does not mean that we have no way of judging between competing ideas of positive health. They too involve theses about *what is*. Their implicit claims about *what should be* and *what can be* are rooted in theories of human nature which, although complex and changeable in its manifestations, consists of real, causally generative mechanisms and is there-fore a knowable aspect of the world. Its discovery has fallen largely to the social sciences and to psychology, encouraged by the development of disciplinary bound-aries to work separately, making unwarranted or at least untheorized assumptions about the object of the other. The crucial meeting-places have been in politics, in discussion of alternative societies; and in psychology, in the theories underlying psychotherapy – in other words, in the theoretical underpinnings of practices aimed at social and individual change. I have chosen to focus on psychotherapy and its ideas of mental health.

If social change is necessary, as argued in Chapter 2, then the institutional-ization of 'normal functioning' ideas of health in the mental health system and other social institutions is itself an aspect of the danger facing human societies. The distinction between what I shall henceforth call health-as-normal-functioning on the one hand and positive health on the other parallels the distinction made in Chapter 2 between the agent as reproducing social structures and the agent as trans-forming them. Because the structural reproductive mechanisms tend to incorporate and modify minor changes (known as 'co-option' by the agents involved), suc-cessful transformative action has to be deliberate and reflexive. It must involve a critique of and rupture with routine social practices and the problematizing of health-as-normal-functioning. For such transformation towards an ecologically sustainable society (accepting here, without argument, the view that existing social structures cannot be adapted to this end), four things have to be true of human nature and therefore of the transformative agents. These raise questions both about what human beings are capable of in general and about what they are capable of in the many particular circumstances of today. However, they are a necessary rather than a sufficient condition of such radical social change.

The first condition concerns human motivation and precludes the psycholo-gical assumptions of rational choice theory and similar reductionist positions. Agents must be capable of the sustained will to change, of envisioning a better society and remaining confident of its possibility and committed to the process of getting there.

Yet this may not be achieved in their lifetime: the major beneficiaries will be their descendants. And this vision, this motivation, have to be achievable *now*, in societies that dangle the dream of instant gratifications in front of us at every turn. The danger is that those who can sustain this motivation do so at the expense of (this particular notion of) positive health. They do not revert to 'normal functioning', but they become rigid. 'The problem . . . is how to act decisively, with the passion that stems from feeling right and good, yet preserve the capacity to be proved wrong' and the flexibility that goes with it (Hoggett, 1992, p. 49). If this cannot be done, the second condition will be breached.

The second condition is that agents be capable of awareness of reality and can put reflexivity at their service to gain the best available knowledge of 'what is'. This, we shall see, is taken as a criterion of health by almost all types of psychotherapy, although their ideas about reality differ. Awareness of reality involves being able to assess the positive possibilities, the real resources of power, as well as the extent and detail of danger. It involves being aware of the emotions, beliefs and impulses we live by. Whether it is possible to function well and effectively in the face of great collective danger, without denying it or suffering disabling anxiety, remains an open question. If it is possible, it probably depends on overcoming isolation so that positive ideas of health, alternative values, are developed within movements aiming at world change.

However, the third condition is that movements have to be built whose internal processes do not sabotage their aims by reproducing the oppressive features of the society they aim to transform. In 1944 Hayek argued that this was impossible (Hayek, 1944, p. 101) and postmodernist thinkers today see it as a chimera (Bauman, 1989, p. 4). Thus the Bolsheviks produced a camp regime which was comparable to that of the tsars, although harsher; the ANC was torn by internal struggles and violence; voluntary organizations often scandalously mistreat their employees. The social change we produce may not be the social change we intended. In part this will depend on how good our information and our analysis are, but processes of scapegoating and exclusion happen in groups which militate against unity and peace (Rowe, 1985, p. 145). Whether political commitment which uses the force of justified anger without acting on hatred and exclusion is possible depends on the strength and flexibility of human social impulses.

A fourth, related, requirement is that we be able to live in the better society we aim to build. As Eastern Europe erupted in 1989, many people attributed the failures of socialism to human nature. 'People simply can't help abusing a "free lunch" society,' they said complacently. If they are right – if the global commons are as certain to be vandalized as the swings in our parks – we are in deep trouble. The question of the causes of sexism, of racism, of the intercommunal divisions that regularly result in atrocities and deaths, is crucial. Would we know how to live in a participatory democracy, whose ecological sustainability depended on our cooperation? Is it a question of changing structures, of educating, of watching until a new generation emerges without our dreadful heritage? Or are we as certain to produce outgroups, to put our greed and desire for comfort above the common good, to prefer present satisfaction to future safety, as we are to breathe, eat and excrete?

These are questions about the natural capacities and tendencies of human beings and their limitations: human nature. Those who deny that any such psychological characteristics exist often forget that a capacity can be universally present without necessarily being realized. Humans can learn to speak, for instance, which is an extraordinarily complex capacity passed down genetically, but if the conditions are not right they will not learn. So in thinking about our current denial of the serious situation which faces us, we have to ask whether some degree of denial is inevitable because of the limitations of our psychic structure, or whether denial is a universal human capacity, socially produced in certain environments. In thinking about the basis of our sociality and our capacity for communal and collective action, we have to look at group processes and group agency and their relationship to what goes on at the individual level.

Is the viciousness that is typical of political action and that frequently sabotages our projects an inherent feature of human nature-in-groups? Last, in thinking about our capacity to live without oppressing others and without acting on greed, we need to reach a conclusion about the psychological mechanisms which produce and reproduce these ways of acting. We need to know whether they are self-generating offshoots of our psychic structure, in other words part of what it means to be human, or whether they are the product of particular – and avoidable – sets of social conditions.

Psychology of this sort is not generally studied in the psychology departments of universities. If anyone addresses these questions, it is psychotherapists, although often without acknowledging their political implications. Chapter 2 argued that sociological theories rest on psychological premises, which are rarely theorized. This chapter has claimed that social explanations bracket assumptions about psychological health, which actually need to be brought into focus and questioned if we are interested in the possibilities of social change. I go on to review in some detail selected influential theories of psychotherapy, in search of psychological theories of the self which can illuminate the scope of human agency and social change.

In the following chapters I shall outline the selected approaches, asking two complex questions of each:

1   What is psychological health? Does it involve an element of social criticism and political activity?

In other words, how does this approach distinguish its notion of positive health from 'health as normal functioning'? Only an approach which provides a critique of and an explanation of denial and conformity is likely to be able to support environmental political projects.

2   What is the relationship between psychic structures and social structures?

How does each contribute to the reproduction of the other and how much scope is there for interrupting this process? Is the approach reductionist, or does it recognize the interdependence of social and psychological structures implied in the duality of structure and agency? In particular, does the theory lead to the conclusion that human beings are collectively capable of halting the trend to environmental destruction, or does it see this trend as rendered inevitable by psychological structures?

Chapter 4

Freud and the inevitability of discontent

Introduction

Freud is popularly considered significant above all because of his emphasis on sex, a view with which Freudians have sometimes colluded (e.g. Jones, 1964, p. 237). Freud himself wrote that a sexual aetiology of the neuroses was 'no new, unheard of proposition' (1962c, p. 149; cf. Ellenberger, 1970, Ch. 7; Symington, 1986, p. 86). Even more fundamental than his theory of infantile sexuality was his emphasis on the causal role of dynamic, intra-psychic processes common to all human beings and irreducible to consciousness and behaviour: what I call in this book human psychological nature. The various schools of psychoanalysis which have emerged during this century differ in their views on these processes and structures. But all follow Freud in agreeing that human psychological nature exists, mediating all human experience. It therefore necessarily plays a causal role in action, social events and social reproduction.

When it came to explaining psychological distress in individuals, Freud's theory also gave a role to constitutional differences (individual differences in the balance and relative weight and strength of the intra-psychic factors) and to external factors including differences in the social environment of different social groups. But these other factors worked *through* intra-psychic factors and it was these that determined the forms their influence could take.

Radicals have plausibly argued that the gradual downgrading of external factors in Freud's theory undermines its original radical promise. This thesis is discussed below. But on the other hand the initial move (largely reneged-on later) from emphasizing constitutional *differences* (what was special about the neurotic) to emphasizing intra-psychic factors *common* to all has enormous radical significance. Freud broke with neurological conceptions of madness, despite his own yearning after physiological reductionism (Jones, 1964, p. 228). He broke with the Enlightenment ideas of madness as lack or loss of reason (Sayers, 1991). Following the great hypnotists and mesmerists of the eighteenth and nineteenth centuries, he established the intelligibility of symptoms of mental distress, undermining the conceptual barrier between mental 'health' and 'illness' and thus giving more potential

The healthy man too is virtually a neurotic ... The difference between nervous health and nervous illness (neurosis) is ... a practical distinction ... how far the person concerned remains capable of a sufficient degree of capacity for enjoyment and active achievement in life. (Freud, 1963, p. 382)

This could but need not imply an equation of health with 'normal functioning'.

Freud's aetiology of illness was based precisely on his aetiology of health. The neurotic was not someone whose mind, like a diseased limb, was not working, but someone whose inner conflicts and attempts at resolution were shared with those of the healthy. Sexuality was not just an important aetiological factor *for those who fell ill* (with the implication that they were of degenerate stock or morally weak). Sexuality played a vital and problematic part in *everyone's* mental life – a contention less stigmatizing for the patient, but more alarming to doctors and the public. In his earliest period Freud also uncovered the common abuse of children, known about yet deliberately not-known (Fromm, 1971, p. 57). Which aspect and which period of his work most disturbed the world has become a hot issue (Masson, 1984, p. 84; Miller, 1985, p. 185; Ellenberger, 1970, p. 440).

Freud's theorization of the unconscious extended the concept of intentionality in a way now generally accepted in Western philosophy and social theory, even by those who reject the key tenets of psychoanalysis. It means that although reasons can still cause actions, our conscious reasons are often mere rationalizations to which we falsely attribute causal status, while our unconsious reasons are by definition unknown to us, the agents, at least at the time. According to Freud, 'rational' and moral considerations have the power to sway us only when they are in tune with unconscious motivations (often represented in consciousness by emotions). The rational is thus rooted in the irrational and the irrational turns out to be intelligible. Freedom of action and concepts of agency in general become far more complicated once we accept the existence of unconscious reasons. One immediate attraction of this sort of complication, however, is that it suggests an explanation of human failure to respond effectively to knowledge of environmental threat.

For my purposes Freud's work can be considered in three periods. These are not chosen for their psychological but for their sociological significance.

1   The Freud of the 'seduction' or 'trauma' theory, the period of collaboration with Breuer, his friendship with Fliess and self-analysis, 1882–1897.
2   The Freud of infantile sexuality and psychodynamics, from the completion of *The Interpretation of Dreams* (1899), through the theoretical shift marked by the 1914 paper 'On Narcissism', up to the end of the First World War.
3   The Freud of the two formulations of the death instinct, in *Beyond the Pleasure Principle* (1920) and *The Ego and the Id* (1923) to his death in 1939. My discussion of (3) focuses on the topographical tripartite structure of mind (with reference to its development by Anna Freud) and Freud's later thinking about the relationship between the psyche and social stru

My exposition aims only to be full enough to allow me to ask and answer the two questions:

1 **What is psychological health?** Can this concept of health ground social criticism? Does it involve an element of political activity?
2 **What is the relationship between social structures and psychological structures?** How do they contribute to each other's reproduction?

The answers to these questions are different in the different periods. My aim is not to discover 'What Freud really thought' but to trace, understand and analyse the recurring concepts and arguments.

From its inception, psychoanalysis has contributed to social criticism by arguing for a greater degree of congruence between social needs and human instinctual satisfaction. At the same time it has been a pessimistic commentator on radical ambitions, arguing that no social change, however radical, can abolish the necessary contradiction between the instinctual drives each individual experiences and the social prohibition on their full satisfaction. I explore this dynamic, which holds the key to Freud's view of the individual/society relationship, through two issues extensively discussed by Freud: disabling 'hysterical' illness and, in a later section, war.

The first Freud: The trauma or seduction theory

Freud's breakdown of the hard and fast division between neurosis and health is the more impressive because his early patients were dramatically ill, though Freud notes that they often seemed cheerful even about disabling symtoms. These patients suffered from hysteria, that ancient disorder which classical medicine had attributed to the literal wanderings of the unsatisfied womb. For centuries it had been treated by administering horrible smells and tastes at the head end to frighten the organ back into its place and pleasant smells and male symbols at the other end to encourage its passage home (Veith, 1965). In the nineteenth century, such practices had given way to prohibitions on masturbation and recommendation of marriage, the transparently punitive injection of ice water into the womb and even clitoridectomy (Showalter, 1987, p. 74).

A sexual aetiology was frequently invoked for various mental disorders of the time. In such complaints as 'neurasthenia' (a vague diagnostic category covering exhaustion, insomnia, headaches, irritability and inability to cope), Freud was in agreement with most of his European colleagues in seeing masturbation, *coitus interruptus* and other forms of inadequate relief of sexual tension as the root cause (Ellenberger, 1970, p. 297). Like them, he prescribed either rest and abstinence or, better, freer heterosexual activity, both for neurasthenia and the 'anxiety neuroses' (which included panic attacks and phobias). It appealed to Freud's materialism to think of the sexual instinct in chemical terms, as a quantitative force which could be transformed but not diminished.

But such views of sexual activity as necessary to mental health could not be readily and simply transferred to women, in whom sexual desire was either denied or pathologized. Hysterics (the vast majority of whom were female) were either seen as debauched or malingerers. Charcot's insistence on hysteria as a *neurological* condition was welcomed by Freud as liberating the hysteric from slander and disrespect. 'The first thing that Charcot's work did was to restore its dignity to the topic. Little by little, people gave up the scornful smile with which the patient could at that time feel certain of being met' (Freud, 1962a, p. 19). This was the view Freud held on his return from Paris in 1886, which shifted during ten years' clinical practice to the view that hysteria was caused by a passive sexual experience before puberty.

The hysteric was someone who had no detectable organic impairment, but was so incapacitated by her symptoms (often including paralysis of the legs or arms) that she had to be cared for. But in the past these women had often been carers themselves and Freud described sick-nursing as playing a significant part in the prehistory of hysteria. Here there is a hint of a social analysis, which is never developed. Elisabeth von R., the fifth case-study in the book, had enjoyed a close relationship with her father, for whom she 'took the place of both a son and a friend with whom he could exchange thoughts. However, it did not escape the father that her psychic constitution deviated from that ideal which one so much desires to see in a girl' (1955a, p. 161). She was argumentative and ambitious. Her father fell ill. Elisabeth nursed him for eighteen months, sleeping in his room and watching over him during the day. A couple of years later she nursed her mother and soon afterwards became ill herself and unable to walk: 'from now on Elisabeth herself became the patient in the family' (1955a, p. 143). Freud's naturalization of gender difference meant that in this and other accounts he only noticed the tiring, emotionally demanding nature of the work, the need to postpone the expression of grief and frustration, to keep the voice lowered and to suppress natural reactions to painful events. He did not link this work of caring with the more general demands on women to give up any notion of independent projects for themselves, although he gives us plenty of evidence of the resulting inner conflict. *This* conflict, fruit of a gendered social environment, has no pathogenic power in Freud's theory. What does have power, but is theoretically unconnected, is a certain sort of early sexual relationship.

Freud's new theory of the sexual aetiology of hysteria sprang from an initial discovery: when his patients were encouraged to trace their symptoms back through free association, they pointed to an 'unbearable idea', which in turn led to an early trauma in the form of sexual abuse. Previous theories had seen the problem as stemming from the sexuality of the sufferer; here it was the sexuality of the abuser on the one hand and the internalized social prohibitions (feelings of shame) on the other which produced the symptoms. In all of his first eighteen cases of hysteria Freud found evidence of premature sexual experience (sexual relationships with other children) or abuse by adults; incidents recounted by the patient 'with the utmost reluctance', eliciting in the recounting 'the most violent sensations' and often continued disbelief in the reality of these memories even as they were most convincingly recollected (1962d, p. 204). In two of his cases the memories had been confirmed as true by other people involved.

Who were the abusers? In both papers on this subject in 1896 it is remarkable that fathers are never mentioned. They speak of sex between children, of whom the older child, a boy, was known or supposed to be the victim of an earlier abuse by a female servant or governess; of isolated assaults by adult strangers; but in the more numerous group 'some adult attendant of the child – a maid, nurse, governess, teacher, unhappily only too often a near relation – initiated the child into sexual intercourse and maintained a regular love-relation with him, often for years, which had its mental counterpart' (Freud, 1962d, p. 208). The father here takes his place in silence, yet we know from Freud's letters to Fliess that the guilt of the father preoccupied his thinking at this time. We also know that in the case of Katherina in *Studies in Hysteria* he substituted an uncle for the father. We also find this poignant footnote concerning another patient:

> I said to her ... that I was quite convinced that ... something else must have happened which she did not mention. She then permitted herself to be drawn into one single allusion, but hardly had she uttered one word when she became mute and her elderly father, sitting behind her, began to sob bitterly. I naturally did not press the patient any further, nor have I ever seen her again. (Freud, 1955a, p. 100)

Why was the event traumatic? For this is not given, as commonsense mistakenly assumes. Freud was tentative about the plausibility of the thesis that 'a premature sexual experience of this kind, undergone by a person whose sex is scarcely differentiated, may become the starting point of a permanent mental abnormality like hysteria' (1962c, p. 153). He was struggling both with the problem of the delayed onset of the supposed effect and with his preconception of the young child as sexually anaesthetic as well as innocent which, ironically, is often used as an excuse by abusers themselves. He concluded that premature sexual stimulation produced little or no effect at the time, but a mental impression of it was reawakened by the sexual development of puberty and only then became pathogenic (Freud, 1962c, p. 154).

However, in one passage Freud refers to the asymetrical power relations between adult and child and the child's dependence on the adult, though he tends to treat both of these as 'natural' and given. He writes with clear feeling about the inherent and immediate harm of such relations:

> All the singular conditions under which the ill-matched pair conduct their love-relations – on the one hand the adult, who cannot escape his share in the mutual dependence necessarily entailed by a sexual relationship, and who is yet armed with complete authority and the right to punish, and can exchange the one role for the other to the uninhibited satisfaction of his moods, and on the other hand the child, who in his helplessness is at the

mercy of this arbitrary will, who is prematurely aroused to every kind of sensibility and exposed to every sort of disappointment, and whose performance of the sexual activities assigned to him is often interrupted by his imperfect control of his natural needs – all these grotesque and yet tragic incongruities reveal themselves as stamped upon the later development of the individual and of his neurosis, in countless permanent effects which deserve to be traced in the greatest detail. (1962d, p. 215)

This does not sound like a sexual experience which was harmless at the time. But Freud never confronted these inconsistencies, nor ever focused directly on the inequality of power as a key factor in transforming 'premature sexual experiences' into abuse. His silences, his inconsistencies, the way 'seduction' and 'abuse' appear side by side without clear differentiation, all pave the way for the replacement of this early account with one which focuses on the agency of the child rather than the adult.

Freud was now advocating a theory of mental illness which in some ways still separated the ill from the well. In this theory, the ill were a group to whom bad things happened – in the external (social) world. They either reacted as any well person would or, for constitutional reasons, overreacted. However, even though the ill were distinguished by the fact that things happened to them which they could not cope with in normal, 'well' ways, their responses remained intelligible and the internal psychic processes which determined those responses were essentially the same as those of well people, although perhaps in certain respects less developed or more intense.

Freud did not consider the idea that bad things were more likely to happen to certain social groups, but did put forward, in these early papers, one clear-cut way in which social structures are implicated in causing psychological distress. Women were more likely to fall ill because they had internalized stronger and more all-embracing prohibitions. 'Such unbearable ideas develop in women chiefly in connection with sexual experiences and sensations . . . a young girl who disapproved of herself because while nursing her sick father she had let her mind dwell on the thought of a young man who had made a slight erotic impression on her' (1962b, p. 48).

Women, then, were more vulnerable to hysteria on two counts: first, more was forbidden them/they forbade themselves more and there is thus more opportunity for conflict. Second, since the specific determinant of hysteria was a premature sexual experience involving passivity: 'we are . . . thus provided with a clue to the reason for the much greater frequency of hysteria in the female sex, which even in childhood is more likely to provoke sexual assaults' (1962f, p. 163). By the same token, in obsessional neurosis where it is a question 'of aggressive acts performed with pleasure and of pleasurable participation in sexual acts . . . this difference . . . explains why the obsessional neurosis appears to favour the male sex' (1962f, p. 168). We have a complex causal picture here involving constitutional differences between the sexes, intra-psychic conflict universal in the human species and the different life events and social expectations for women and men.

Class, too, could affect your vulnerability. If you belonged to a group (such as the working class) which internalized less strong prohibitions, even ideas which caused conflict would be more likely to remain available (see the case of Katherina in *Studies*). 'Since the ego's attempt at defence depends upon the whole moral and intellectual development of the person concerned, the fact that hysteria is so much rarer in the lower classes than would follow from its specific aetiology is no longer entirely incomprehensible' (1962d, p. 211). Here too the causal role of the social environment is mediated through intra-psychic processes and vice versa, but its significance is plain.

The social environment was responsible for much inner conflict. More freedom about sexuality, more opportunity for sexual satisfaction, less hypocrisy and fewer prohibitions would promote better mental health. Freud did not discuss the preconditions for getting rid of or minimizing child abuse, but there is a clear implication that if there were less of it there would be less mental illness. To this extent, Freud did believe that social structures were implicated in bringing about psychological distress. But what was his early idea of mental health?

Freud's first aim was to free his patients from their disabling presenting problems. He constantly emphasized the serious nature of neurotic illness, with its worst case outcome of incapacity for life (1962e, p. 284). Even without social reform, if inner conflict could be experienced and worked through consciously, although psychic pain must result, there would be no illness. The early cathartic theory and the notion of preventive abreaction suggested that the expression of emotions was an aspect of mental health, but this was in contrast to the containment and stoicism which was Freud's own style and has become part of the culture of psychoanalysis. Even while praising a woman who worked through painful experiences thoroughly and regularly, Freud seemed uncomfortable and obliged to reassure us that she was not ill (1955a, p. 164). He was not yet sure whether repression (as he was beginning to call it) could ever be healthy and whether 'successful defence' was health, or merely 'apparent health' (1962f, p. 169). In 1895 he described the aim of his treatment as 'transforming your hysterical misery into common unhappiness' (1955a, p. 305). Mental health was, then, the freest possible conscious access to the mind; the capacity to bear all ideas, to face them and consciously to decide how best to act.

The second Freud: Infantile sexuality and psychic reality

The *Interpretation of Dreams*, Freud's favourite of his books, marks the shift from the 'seduction' theory to the theory of infantile sexuality (Freud, 1953a). During Freud's 'self-analysis', with Fliess as analyst *in absentia*, he moved from the fear that his father would turn out to have been an abuser, to the belief (after his father's death) in his own incestuous wishes towards his father, jealous hatred of his mother and fear of punishment. By 1899 he had definitely come to the conclusion that hysterics and other neurotics suffered not from 'reminiscences' but from repressed wishes, expressed in unconscious fantasies which he had mistaken for memories of actual events. These fantasies sprang from the child's own incestuous wishes towards their first love objects, the parents; and the wish to get rid of the parent of the same sex so as to have the other to themselves. At first Freud saw these wishes as a product of puberty projected back on to infancy. But gradually (Jones, 1964, p. 279) he moved from the position that infants and young children were sexually anaesthetic as well as sexually innocent to the position that their ardent and ultimately forbidden desires fuelled both neuroses and normal development.

The dynamics of unconscious processes were theorized in this second period as never before. *The Interpretation of Dreams* (1900) was the first of Freud's works to distinguish between the pleasure principle (the tendency to seek wish fulfilment, if necessary hallucinated) and the reality principle (which modified unconscious wishes and accepted substitutes in order to get some wishes fulfilled in reality); between the unconscious thinking which ignored logic and time and the 'secondary process' thinking of the conscious mind. He understood dreams as energized by repressed wishes which arouse sleep-disturbing anxiety. The dreamer, caught between the urgency of the wish and the anxiety resulting from its forbidden nature, allowed it expression in a compromise form, distorted and condensed. *The Psychopathology of Everyday Life* (1905) similarly analysed slips of the tongue (Freud, 1960). Both books concentrated on well people and emphasized that the processes involved in the formation of these ordinary 'symptoms' were exactly the same as those involved in neurosis (1953a, p. 569).

In 1905, in *Three Essays on the Theory of Sexuality*, Freud described the construction of adult genital heterosexuality from several primary drives (Freud, 1953b). Once again 'abnormality' ('perversion' and 'inversion') were theorized in terms of normal processes. A constitutional difference between the well and the neurotic remained part of the theory, but it was by no means hard and fast: 'an unbroken chain bridges the gap between the neuroses in all their manifestations and normality . . . we are all to some extent hysterics . . . the disposition to perversions . . . must form a part of what passes as the normal constitution' (1953b, p. 171). *Three Essays* theorized the development of the child's love for the mother as rooted in the sexual instinct, which is initially linked to the taking-in of nourishment. The affection between parents and child is described as 'damped down libido' (1953b, p. 223). The sexual drive, constructed out of primitive components, is the *essence* of love. Its opposite is not aggression (which is a reversal) but self-preservation. The Unconscious is the source of libido as well as the unstable prison of the repressed. The Conscious mind, a self-preserving filter, allows unconscious impulses through in modified or symbolic form, provided there is a socially acceptable place for them.

In the case-study of 'Little Hans' (1909) Freud described how a little boy's fear of castration by his father in retribution for his sexual love for his mother resulted in a phobia of horses: the triangular dynamics he had discerned in himself in his self-analysis (1955b). He saw the Oedipus situation as timeless, produced by the biologically given structure of the human family and of the developmental tasks facing the child. This normal problem could only be solved through the risky process of repression, which was both the root of neurosis *and* a necessary defence in normal psychic life.

The aetiological role of social structures

> Freud's interpretation – that the sexual violence that so affected the lives of his women patients was nothing but fantasy – posed no threat to the existing social order. Therapists could thus remain on the side of the successful and the powerful, rather than of the miserable victims of family violence. (Masson, 1984, p. xxii)

> Freud's abandonment of the seduction theory was a victory for common sense and the beginning of a new era, one in which it became possible to elucidate the way in which fantasies can distort memory and in which infantile sexual wishes and parental attitudes combine to generate what we now call the Oedipus complex. (Rycroft, 1984, p. 3)

An interesting aspect of the transition which gave birth to psychoanalysis proper became a *cause célèbre* in the mid-1980s. Freud was accused by Masson, a brand-new analyst and protégé of the great, of backing away from the trauma theory for fear of the implication that his own father was an abuser, thus beginning 'a trend away from the real world that . . . is at the root of the present-day sterility of psychoanalysis and psychiatry throughout the world' (Masson, 1984, p. 144). Masson's attacks were dismissed as 'acting out', but their substance was more soberly considered in feminist circles, along with Miller's parallel arguments (1983).

Certainly, in these 15 or so years Freud's view of sexuality in the aetiology of the neuroses had definitively changed, placing far more emphasis on constitutional differences affecting the working of intra-psychic mechanisms. The assertion of the importance of fantasy weakened the role of external events and therefore of social structures as causal factors. What made some events traumatic was their relationship to the person's unconscious fantasy life.

'Psychic reality' was to be taken into account 'alongside practical reality' (Freud, 1957a, p. 17). This shift has been hailed as a great advance on several counts. Some have argued that only causal theories at the level of intra-psychic processes, the properly psychological, could consolidate Freud's demolition of the barrier between the 'healthy' and the 'ill'. In that case the theory of infantile sexuality has the advantage, for the earlier theory 'had the effect of sharply separating the personal history and the psychic characteristics of the mentally ill from the world of normal mental development, thereby blocking the way to a more general and unified concept of mental activity' (McGrath, 1986, p. 194). A simple monocausal 'external events' explanation of mental illness really would do this, a problem we come back to in discussing radical theories under the heading of 'the deficit model' (see Chapter 8).

But we shall see that the movement away from external and social factors involves a similar danger. For explanations cannot only be at the level of intra-psychic factors, which are common to all: they must also imply that those who fall ill are either inherently different, treated differently or both. The movement away from environmental factors inevitably brought constitutional predispositions to neurosis back to the forefront.

Defenders of the shift claim that the early theory was based on a simple, Humean model of causation as constant conjunction, so that a 'real event' such as sexual abuse was *invariably* followed by trauma and illness. This ignores the fact that in the 'seduction theory' Freud already had a dynamic concept of illness as a defence, as one of a repertoire of *responses*. Scott and others are right to say that no events are intrinsically traumatic, since it is not the event but its (mediated) effect on the person which is at issue (Scott, 1988, p. 91). However, a theory of psychic development may well conclude that because of the way humans are, some events will always tend to be harmful to them, even though their exact effect cannot be predicted. Freud's elaboration of intra-psychic processes, including fantasy, enriched the theory, but something was lost. This was the recognition that social relations of power affect both what happens in sexual relations between people and also the *meaning* of those relations. Since how events are experienced is a function of their meaning, power relations must be relevant to the potential pathogenic impact of certain forms of sexual relations.

Freud did not initially believe that his early patients' stories were entirely the result of fantasy. He thought that by chance his patients had included an unusually high frequency of cases of abuse (1953d, p. 274), but he was already mentioning the difficulty of distinguishing memory and fantasy. Eventually he came to believe that such early sexual experiences played a pathogenic role because they coincided with forbidden wishes, which had in any case to be defended against. At the most the experience acted to intensify the conflict. Increasingly Freud came to see the stories of sexual 'seduction' as unconsciously motivated, as actually made up 'to cover up the autoerotic activity of the first years of childhood' (1957a, p. 17). In 1915 he wrote that while seduction did sometimes occur:

> it is still not as often real as it seemed at first from the results of analysis. Seduction by children of the same age or older is more frequent than by adults; and when girls who bring forward this event in the story of their childhood regularly introduce the father as the seducer, neither the phantastic character of this accusation nor the motive actuating it can be doubted. (1963, p. 370)

Children's 'nearest male relatives' did sometimes abuse them, Freud went on, but such occurrences 'belonged to the later years of childhood and had been transposed to an earlier time' (ibid.). Even here something stopped Freud naming the father as a real abuser.

In *On the History of the Psychoanalytical Movement*, also written about 1914, Freud described children as sometimes both exaggerating and provoking sexual experiences, citing Abraham's 1907 paper as the 'last word' on this subject (Freud, 1957a, p. 18). In that paper Abraham argued that when seduction of children by adults does occur, children who are constitutionally predisposed to neurosis will be easily bribed with presents or sweets, will fail to defend themselves 'actively and in earnest' and will sometimes 'quite definitely provoke adults in a sexual manner' (Abraham, 1942, p. 48). He drew a clear analogy with the way in which women 'provoke rape'. Children's silence reflected their feelings of guilt for their compliance, he wrote. He ignored the conflict arising in cases where the abuser is well-known to the child, preferring to assume that the abuser is a stranger and that the child is old enough to resist. Freud agreed that some people produce the external events required by their psychic development, whether this be normal or neurotic. 'Childhood experiences of this kind (i.e. sexual ones) are in some way necessarily required by the neurosis. If they can be found in real events, well and good, but if reality has not supplied them they will be evolved out of hints and elaborated by fantasy. The effect is the same' (1963, p. 370).

From environmental aetiology we have now returned, via intra-psychic processes, to a new version of the demonology of the neurotic, whose indefatigable constitution moulds experience to the shape the illness requires. The power dimension Freud once recognized was now obscured. Take the Dora case, for instance. Dora was brought to Freud by her father, who had his own ideas of a 'healthy outcome' of her hysteria – one that would allow him to continue his relationship with his friend's wife without Dora's interference. Herr K, Dora's father's friend, got her alone by a pretext and kissed her on the lips. Dora felt a sensation of disgust (1953c, p. 28). Freud writes: 'the behaviour of this child of fourteen was already entirely and completely hysterical. I should without question consider a person hysterical in whom an occasion for sexual excitement elicited feelings that were preponderately or exclusively unpleasurable' (ibid.). He goes on to refer to the 'genital sensation which would certainly have been felt by a healthy girl in such circumstances' (ibid.).

Many interpretations of Freud's interpretation have been made. What matters here is his failure to see the relevance of the inequality of power between Dora and Herr K and Dora's general powerlessness to her response.[1] Freud may be right to suggest that Dora repressed any sexual feelings she had at that moment. But in his puzzlement he seems blind to the 'tragic incongruities' operating here, to the power differential to which, in other adult-child couples, he once drew attention as a possible source of that repression. Herr K's behaviour is unquestioned, as if appropriate, while Dora's is 'hysterical'. The concept of 'abuse', which lurked untheorized behind the 'seduction theory', has now completely gone. External events are understood entirely in terms of libido, despite the place given in the theory to the self-preservative instincts. The difference between a real and a fantasized sexual relation with a parent-figure is in terms of the strength of instinctual demands and the person's readiness to handle it.

This is why, despite the relative theoretical meagreness of the trauma theory, some critics of psychoanalysis hark back to it. Since 1979 Alice Miller, a Swiss psychoanalyst, has been writing about various forms of child abuse. She argues that ever since the turn away from the trauma theory, psychoanalysis has been colluding with the socially sanctioned abuse of the child.[2]

> Not long ago, charges were brought against a man in Switzerland who took each of his six children to the woods when they were four years old (in the Oedipal stage!) and performed anal intercourse with them. Probably the same thing had been done to him at that age. We can only hope that if a son of his should someday require analysis he will not be told ... that the scenes he is describing represent his 'homosexual fantasies'. (Miller, 1985, p. 43)

Even if the analyst merely says that it makes no difference whether reality or fantasy is involved here, the patient will still not be able to comprehend his anger because the analyst has not acknowledged its validity.

> The roots of neurosis lie in the enforced repression not of the child's so-called instinctual drives but of his or her awareness of having been traumatised and in the prohibition against articulating this, which was internalised at a very early age ... Cruelty on the part of the parents is always interpreted as the product of the child's drive fantasies, generated by the child's own cruelty. (ibid., p. 216)

Miller's critique illuminates an important aspect of Freud's notion of mental health, which was part of his legacy to psychoanalysis. While sadism was recognized as one of the component sexual instincts, anger – especially appropriate, reactive anger rather than hatred – remained untheorized in psychodynamic theory.

Mental health in the dynamic theory

To try to sum up the second period is inevitably to do an injustice to the continual movements in Freud's thought as he kept trying new ways of conceptualizing the relationship between the ego and the drives. The most important of these shifts was the 1914 essay 'On Narcissism' in which Freud tentatively extended the idea of two types of instincts, sexual and non-sexual (self-preserving), which initially run along the same tracks (in breast-feeding) and eventually diverge. The key to healthy development is the move in which the infant, who originally loves him/herself (auto-erotism), makes his first carer his earliest sexual object (anaclitic object choice). In this theory inner conflict results not only from a clash of sexual and non-sexual instincts, but also from the reproaches of the ego-ideal, the (approved) part of the self which the adult continues to love and which is internal spokesperson for the parents and society (Freud, 1957b, p. 96). This theoretical development was superseded, but one of its residues was the idea that mental health involves loving yourself realistically: enough (self-esteem), but not too much. Parental adoration of their children is not (as some humanists and radicals would have it) a recognition of their true nature, but a disguised regression to their own unbridled narcissism: a massive over-valuation (Freud, 1957b, p. 91).

Unsurprisingly, Freud's idea of mental health in this second period was not uniform. On the one hand, in describing sexuality as constructed he robbed heterosexual genital sex of its straightforwardly 'natural' status, allowing Marcuse to advocate the embrace of polymorphous perversity as part of the abolition of 'surplus repression' (Marcuse, 1972, p. 145). On the other hand, Freud's description of illness as a pseudo-satisfaction to replace genuine but frustrated erotic needs legitimized Reich's panacea of universal genitality (Reich, 1951). In general, Freud suggested that the key to mental health was to minimize repression (Freud, 1955b, p. 123). Where repression failed, psychoanalysis could lift it to allow the psychical conflict to reach a better outcome. Through making the Unconscious conscious, its wishes could be wholly or partly granted, sublimated (diverted to a 'higher' and socially acceptable aim) or brought under conscious control and rejected. But throughout this period there are also references to *successful* repression as the acme of mental health. Healthy people are those 'in whom the repression of unconscious impulses has on the whole been quite successful' (1957a, p. 28). Indeed, the *Three Essays* describe repression as 'organically determined' and as necessary for the development of the species to a higher civilization (1953b, pp. 177, 242), all prolegomena to the theme of Freud's third, post-1914 period.

The road to mental health lay in recognizing and accepting (or consciously rejecting) one's own wishes and one's own responsibility. As far as the exigencies of the external world went, mental health involved either stoical acceptance or – where possible – active steps to master the environment. Knowing when acceptance rather than resistance was appropriate required the ability to think clearly, which was threatened by the necessity of repression. Overall the ideal was then to keep repression to a minimum: to allow the greatest development of our mental powers, however uncomfortable and difficult this might be.

The death instinct and the origins of morality

How do we imagine the process by which an individual attains to a higher plane of morality? The first answer is sure to be: he is good and noble from his very birth, his very earliest beginnings. We need not consider this any further. (Freud, 1957c, p. 281)

Beyond the Pleasure Principle was written in 1919 and drew on Freud's clinical experience of wartime trauma as well as his own pain and disillusion. The 'pleasure principle' could not explain the obsessive repetition of unpleasant events, by dreaming, by children's play and by 'acting out' in waking life. In the late Freud, overwhelming anxiety should lead to repression and forgetting, rather than the repetitive representation of painful events. Freud's short book reads like a conversation with himself, a conversation about the relationship between the self-preservative and erotic instincts (are all instincts sexual at root?), about human drives towards life and death. He raises possibilities only to reject them, but he does reach the firm conclusion that there is a death instinct. At one point he hypothesizes that all instincts seek to restore an earlier state of affairs and the earliest state of affairs is: the inanimate. It follows that the aim of all life is death. Our self-preservative instincts struggle to keep us alive simply to ensure that each organism follows its own path to death (1955d, p. 39).

This gloomy speculation puzzled and worried Freud's colleagues and never became part of developed psychoanalytic theory. The death instinct *did* find a future in its own right as Thanatos, opposed by Eros, in the later tripartite theory. But for our purposes *Beyond the Pleasure Principle* is of special interest. Like 'On Narcissism', it tries to situate human beings in the context of the emergence of the organic from the inorganic. Its 'grand narrative' is so grand that it is hard to describe it merely as 'implausible'; at this level we could hardly recognize plausibility. But it has some resonance in our current epoch, when we seem to be witnessing the return of the organic to the inorganic as a result of human practices whose consequences are fairly well understood, yet which are continually reproduced.

Whether as a result of defeatism or of mature intellectual development, Freud settled on the conception of the tripartite mind described in *The Ego and the Id* (Freud, 1961a). His daughter (and North American ego psychology) inherited and developed this less fluid, less ambiguous model. Psychic conflict was no longer between unconscious and conscious parts of the mind, but between the life and death instincts – both unconscious – and between the id, ego and superego, of which only parts of the ego are conscious. The original psyche is the id, a turbulent pool of instinctual wishes into which repressed ideas are hurled like fallen angels. From this great sink first ego, then superego become differentiated. The ego's hard task is to fulfil at least some id-impulses in whatever feasible modified form is acceptable to the superego, representative of society and its demands.

The superego is formed when the boy resolves the Oedipus complex by identifying with his father and renouncing his incestuous love for his mother. But in girls, who experience themselves as already castrated, the Oedipus complex tends to tail-off rather than become resolved and fear of social shame and loss of love replace the threat of castration. The result is a weaker, less firmly internalized superego in women, so that the precepts of civilization are in some respects less tolerable to them than to men (Freud, 1961c, p. 103). For boys and men, then, and to a lesser extent for women, the superego is the precipitate of the father's (society's) disapproval, charged with castration anxiety. It takes on the aggressive, destructive nature of the death instinct (including the child's anger with the parents at having to forego instinctual satisfactions). It constantly monitors and criticizes·

the poor ego [which] serves three severe masters, and does
to bring their claims and demands into harmony with one an(

claims are always divergent and often seem incompatible. No wonder that the ego often fails in its task. Its three tyrannical masters are the external world, the superego and the id. (Freud, 1964, p. 77)

Hemmed in on all sides, the ego reacts with anxiety. When other means of dealing with painful anxiety fail, the ego may resort to forming a symptom, a symbolic or hallucinatory wish fulfilment which will quiet the roarings of the wolf within but is sufficiently disguised to satisfy the superego. Illness is just another way of coping with the profound antagonism between human beings and human society.

Civilization and renunciation

Civilisation . . . is built up on the suppression of instincts. Each individual has surrendered some part of his possessions – some part of the sense of omnipotence or the aggressive . . . inclinations in his personality. From these contributions has grown civilisation's common possession of material and ideal property. Besides the exigencies of life, no doubt it has been family feelings, derived from erotism, that have induced the separate individuals to make this renunciation . . . a progressive one in the evolution of civilisation. (Freud, 1959, p. 187)

Freud recognized society as a human creation, one that we created and continue to create with the best of ourselves. Yet he reiterated that it is our enemy, identifying the self with the id, which 'expresses the true purpose of the individual organism's life' (Freud, 1955g, p. 148). The id exists *before* the other agencies and in this sense Freud saw the individual as predating the social self. This primitive self is forced to renounce instinctual satisfactions under the aegis of the ego, which recognizes the increased chance, in an ordered society, of getting some wishes fulfilled and living to tell the tale. In *Civilisation and its Discontents* Freud focuses on the high price we have to pay for civilization. Civilization has to restrict sexual life, so as to allow a predictable, orderly society without endless fights. Genital love, gone as soon as sated, must be transformed into more lasting, less exclusive affection (1961c, p. 102). The energy thus diverted can be invested in culture, not only in aim-inhibited love (affection) but also in the sublimations represented by science and art. Civilization has to require us to do the impossible: to love our fellow citizens, even those we do not know or have reason to suspect or dislike. Only the existence of an outgroup – other nations, ethnic minorities and so on – makes this civilized 'love' possible, hence the inevitability of war (1961c, p. 115) and the impossibility, one would have thought, of international cooperation to halt environmental destruction. The things we value in civilization are the products of Love: its order, its esteem for the intellect, its regulation of social relationships. But they are held in place by Death: by the aggressive instinct which the superego draws on in its persecution of the good citizen (1961c, p. 129).[3]

Reason and the civilizing process are derivatives of Eros, the life-instinct: aim-inhibited, unifying love. The omnipresence of the death instinct and the danger of reversion to Eros' genital form mean that social solidarity rests on shaky foundations. This becomes apparent in periods of crisis and war. Nevertheless, Freud and the psychoanalytic community believed that, in the long run, civilization was an inexorable process. In 1918 the Ferenczi expressed their enduring hopes for humanity and the victory of culture:

> Regarded *sub specie* psychoanalysis, the recent frightful events fall into place as merely episodes in a still very primitive social organisation. And even if our hopes deceive us and mankind remain the victim of their unconscious to the very end, still we have been vouchsafed a glimpse behind the scenes, and knowledge of the truth can compensate us for . . . much suffering. (Jones, 1953, p. 7)

Sociologically, Freud was an evolutionist who shared the racism of the day in his identification of civilization with European societies. He was also a Lamarckian, believing in the genetic inheritance of acquired characteristics. Our ancestors' sacrifice allows us to inherit a (slight) 'tendency . . . towards transmutation of egoistic into social instincts' (1957c, p. 298). We in our turn must renounce aggression and much direct sexual satisfaction in favour of aim-inhibited, social concern. The process is fragile and unsteady, but sure. 'The voice of the intellect is a soft one, but it does not rest until it has gained a hearing . . . This is one of the few points on which one may be optimistic about the future of mankind' (Freud, 1961b, p. 53).

In a polemic against historical materialism, Freud asserted the independence of this civilizing tendency:

> we must not forget that the mass of mankind, subjected though they are to economic necessities, are borne on by a process of cultural development – some call it civilisation – which is no doubt influenced by all the other factors, but which is equally certainly independent of them in its origin; it is comparable to an organic process, and is quite capable of itself having an effect on the other factors . . . the progressive strengthening of the scientific spirit seems to be an essential part of it. (1964, p. 179)

In the long run, Love will hold Death at bay. The intellect, as an aspect of Eros, exerts a unifying influence on people. Its erotic origins guarantee that reason 'would not fail to concede to human emotions . . . the position to which they are entitled . . . [Reason] would prove to be the strongest unifying force among men, and would prepare the way for future unifications (1964, p. 219).[4]

This, then, is Freud's greatest hope for society, for the general attainment of mental health in the form of the domination of thinking, aimed at minimizing human suffering. Such an outcome – and perhaps only such an outcome – would be adequate to meet the environmental threat described in Chapter 2. But the domination of thinking is not the whole of Freud's conception of psychological health, nor is it easily attained.

Psychological health: The view from ego-psychology

In Freud's later theory, psychological health entailed the domination of the ego, the site of reason. The aim of analysis must be 'to strengthen the ego, to make it more independent of the superego, to widen its field of vision, and so extend its organisation that it can take over new portions of the id. Where id was, there shall ego be. It is reclamation work' (1964, p. 80).

There are two puzzling aspects of this conception of mental health. First, Freud's conception of the ego which, like a skin, is turned towards reality and tries to modify the id's demands so that they can be met within the conditions of the real world. But if the 'shoulds' of the superego are to be given up because their aggressive, guilt-inducing force is more productive of neurosis than health, does this mean that the liberated ego is inherently prosocial, rather than simply selfishly reality-oriented? Freud seems to be teetering here towards the humanistic view that the conscious self, if untrammelled by the past and by guilt, is naturally good – just as he believes that the domination of thought will naturally lead to the aim of reducing human suffering. Other readings are possible. It could be that the ego recognizes conformity to socially accepted mores as expedient. It could be that because thought arises from the sublimation of erotic drives, it retains a unifying tendency. Most likely of all, the weakening of the superego (the negative side of conscience) need not entail any corresponding weakening of the ego-ideal. Whatever Freud meant by it, ego-psychology's theory of the 'conflict-free zone' of the ego came to occupy this ambiguous space.

The second puzzling aspect concerns the relationship between this notion of health and the earlier view of analysis as bringing repressed material into consciousness, recovering hidden memories, with psychological health being the capacity to face up to this newly uncovered material and deal with it. In the tripartite theory, analysis does not so much seek to lift repressions in general as to review them, lifting some and reconstructing others so that they are equal to a heavier strain and are not in conflict with the ego (Freud, 1955f, p. 227). In this we already see the conflict between truth and defence which bedevils the ego-psychological conception of health. In Anna Freud's classic work *The Ego and the Mechanisms of Defence* (1937), the defences appear both as necessary protections for the ego and as obscuring its grasp of reality and therefore limiting agency. Her biologism is more straightforward than her father's. The instincts are biological. The ego is an emergent social level in constant danger of reversion to its id-origins and fearing annihilation in the face of overwhelmingly strong urges. This fear, as well as the fear of external sanctions, result in anxiety which leads infants to mobilize defences. Their choice of defence determines their future personality. Some of the defences Anna Freud describes are highly relevant to the denial of environmental crisis (Freud, A., 1937).

Denial in fantasy (as in makebelieve play) is normal in children. For adults it can be more difficult to tell ourselves compensatory daydreams because of the mature ego's need for synthesis. As long as children remain in touch with reality most of the time, we allow them to pretend they have an imaginary friend or (like little Hans) a grown-up penis. Such pretence can obviate the need for more permanent defensive measures. Anna Freud describes flight, or avoidance of painful situations, as a comparable measure in adults, in whom it tends to become a permanent restriction. This must surely be one of the commonest coping mechanisms, especially with regard to unpleasant facts like global warming. Many of us can function well as long as we keep our minds off certain painful and threatening subjects: a 'prophylaxis' which, according to Anna Freud, the ego undertakes 'at its peril' (1937, p. 112), because it restricts the ability to think.

Some responses to instinctual danger are neither neurotic nor ego-restricting. Sublimation, the transformation of the instincts into socially acceptable forms, allows their actual satisfaction (Freud, A., 1937, p. 56). Writing a thesis or painting a picture can replace erotic pleasure. The development of the intelligence plays a similar role as a response to instinctual danger, but shades into a defence in the intellectualization which Anna Freud describes as typical of adolescence (1937, p. 174). The defences proper (against both the instincts and the feelings they evoke) are necessarily two-edged tools. Displacement of a feeling on to someone else (as when a child hates another woman instead of her mother) means a distortion of the perception of reality and could lead to trouble. Turning aggression against the self can protect others but makes you feel appalling. Projecting feelings on to others similarly distances you from reality. Somatic conversion is clearly uncomfortable. Isolation (splitting-off a feeling or urge from the rest of mental life) requires some keeping up and obviously interferes with thought, since various associations become prohibited. Undoing (a compulsive attempt to reverse some action of the subject's which is felt to have been harmful) is not always possible and, in so far as it is compulsive, remains self-deceptive. As for repression, the original and most powerful defence mechanism, it requires a lot of energy to keep in place and most dangerously it can destroy the integrity of the personality (1937, p. 54).

Yet Anna Freud obviously thinks defences compatible with normality and essential to the development of sociality and cooperative life. She went more fully into the question of the necessity of defence in *Normality and Pathology in Childhood* (1966b), where she argued for the necessity of the superego. Even though too strict a superego breeds neurosis, the child has to internalize social rules – first those of the parents and later those of the community – to achieve 'adaptation to a community of adults' (Freud, A., 1966b, p. 183). 'What a functioning superego is expected to ensure is not the individual's identification with the content of any specific laws but his acceptance and internalisation of the existence of a governing norm in general' (ibid.). Whereas in 1936 Anna Freud focused on the distress and pain of socialization, 30 years later she focuses more on the use of defence to enable individuals to adapt to society while retaining some flexibility and capacity for enjoyment. The socializing processes, while protecting the child against potentially delinquent tendencies, 'also restrict, inhibit and impoverish his original nature' (Freud, A., 1966b, p. 177). But this cannot be helped, since development is twofold:

> The strengthening of the ego and its defensive organisation is itself an essential part of the child's growth and comparable in importance to the unfolding and maturing of the drives. The real antithesis is rooted ... in the aims of development themselves, namely, full individual freedom (implying free drive activity) versus compliance with social norms (implying drive restraint). (ibid.)

Defence is no longer seen as something which must be minimized in the service of psychological health, so as not to interfere with the dominance of reason and intellect in the ego and its capacity for rational agency (including for social change). Adaptation to society has become the key aspect of health: resolving the contradiction in Freud's notion.

In her emphasis in adaptation Anna Freud was influenced by her old colleague and brother in analysis, Heinz Hartmann (both were analysed by Sigmund Freud). His famous monograph *Ego Psychology and the Problem of Adaptation* is based on a set of lectures he delivered in Vienna in 1937. Hartmann aimed to transform psychoanalysis into a general psychology, arguing that the ego is a whole system of functions, not all of which are (normally) involved in conflict with the drives. He stipulated a 'conflict-free sphere' of ego functioning, which included thinking as well as aspects of perception, intention, language, memory and motor development – and thus earned Lacan's title of 'cherub of psychoanalysis'. Adaptation became the main criterion of psychological wellbeing. 'Generally speaking, we call a man well adapted if his productivity, his ability to enjoy life and his mental equilibrium are undisturbed' (Hartmann, 1958, p. 23). Ego-psychology has been the butt of radical critiques for its emphasis on 'adjustment to reality' as the criterion of health and aim of therapy. Mannoni, for instance, accuses it of seeing the patient as an immigrant who has to be acculturated, with psychoanalysis as a tool of the great 'melting pot' (1971, p. 183). Indeed, there is something disturbing about Hartmann's words, with their complete failure to specify the social context in which such equilibrium would be appropriate.

Hartmann offers a bridge to humanistic psychology with its 'true self'. But where humanistic psychology uses the 'true self' to found social criticism, Hartmann's picture is a relativist one. He sees his relativism as progressive, as a blow against dogmatism (1964, p. 14). We are back with health as normal functioning, which will depend on social context: 'individual propensities which amount to disturbances of adaptation in one social group ... may fulfil a socially essential function in another' (Hartmann, 1964, p. 32). The only limit on relativism is the concept of the 'average expectable environment', which includes the whole range of environments which somehow or other provide the minimum preconditions for development. This formulation at least allows for the possibility that some environments cannot be adapted to, as Anna Freud knew well from her work in war nurseries and with child survivors of Therienstadt (1966a). Nevertheless, this limiting concept tends to focus on the micro-social, the family, rather than any wider oppressive aspects of the culture: 'the average expectable environment is foremost the mother and her maternal needs which reciprocate the infant's needs. Behind the mother stand her husband, the concept of family, and the entire social structure (Blanck and Blanck, 1974, p. 28).

Hartmann, who found refuge from Nazism in the USA, did recognize that for some people actual fighting or fleeing, rather than their defensive 'psychical cor- relates', are the best forms of adaptation (Van Der Leeuw, 1971, p. 56). In his early monograph, although he describes social structure as the aspect of exernal reality to which 'man' has most need to adapt, Hartmann emphasizes that adaptation does not always involve changing the self. 'Alloplastic adaptation' (changing the environ- ment) is equally valid. 'We know, for instance, that not all people can tolerate full compliance with the external world and its demands (for example, social demands)' (Hartmann, 1958, p. 54). In other words, conformity can cause unbearable distress – although he detracts from the potential radical power of this statement by mak- ing it sound like a weakness of individuals ('I just can't stand being constantly discriminated against'). He can encompass individually motivated social change, but not such concepts as justice and oppression. If required to distinguish on health grounds between the adaptive response of the slave who stays on the plantation, accepts society's view of who she is and looks to the few satisfactions slavery allows and the slave who risks her life by running away, he might prefer the former. (Specific external situations, Hartmann says, may require responses which intern- ally limit the person (Hartmann, 1964, p. 16).) We are, after all, programmed to adapt to reality: that is the destiny of the ego.

The theoretical tension implicit in Freud's tripartite theory is thus just as acute in the work of Anna Freud and later ego-psychological revisionists such as Hartmann. Is health the recognition of truth, the ability to live with a clear-sighted if uncom- fortable view of both the reality of the inner world – what we really want – and that of the outer world – what is really happening? Or does health lie in successful social functioning, reliant on minimizing pain through the use of defence mechan- isms which downgrade the value and possibility of reality testing? There is a tension between two sets of values in ego-psychology: the idea of normality as constructed through a set of wise and appropriate defences, which protect from psychic pain with the minimum distortion of judgement and memory, and the idea of a clear-seeing conflict-free zone of the ego which needs no defence.

Ego-psychology thus contains an intriguing paradox. The ego, when free of conflict, is a clear window on truth. The analyst's job is to enlarge this window and assist the patient to clean, or even remove, the dirty glass. However, part of the vista that can be seen from the window is distressingly unpleasant and may set up internal conflict which prevents normal functioning. In this case the analyst's job may be to help the patient replace the part of the glass from which this nasty view can be seen, with an opaque softening or distorting pane. Some people are so easily disturbed that they want their whole window opaque. This will necessarily limit their information about the world and thus their functioning. On this naïve realist view truth seems very accessible: the clear screen in no way dims our vision. Yet adaptation to society, normal social functioning, is valued above truth as a therapeutic aim.

To return to Freud. In his pessimistic conception of human nature we are condemned to desire what we can never have – not only because it is forbidden, but because it is inherently unattainable and illusory. Mental health must involve giving up our desires in accordance with reality, but the brutal way in which we do this – through defence mechanisms which hide our desires even from ourselves – in turn threatens mental health by getting us out of touch with reality. Ideally, we should come to accept our desires (the id) while intellectually recognizing them as undesirable and unattainable. The continuing need for the defences is rooted in the difficulty of this: few women are capable of consciously recognizing and repudiating the residue of their desire to be men; few man can face up to their enduring fear of castration (Freud, 1955f, p. 252). So mental health must be a compromise, in which the ego dominates the personality structure and has a realistic vision of both the desires it mediates and of the requirements of social life.

In trying to reach this compromise, the ego looks for the best possible conditions in the external world. Freud's concept of mental health therefore does include the project of changing society to increase the chances of human happiness. However, such attempts are not compatible with mental health when:

1 the aspect of the social structure people are attempting to change is unchangeable because it is based on human nature itself (this would rule out much of feminism);
2 the wish to change society in particular aspects is a cover for general, instinctual hostility to civilization as such (deep ecology at its most misanthropic?); and
3 the wish to right particular wrongs is linked with a stultifying illusion, comparable to religion, such as the Marxist belief that people are naturally good and only culturally evil.

Psychic processes and social structures

Since illness is a response to the terrible anxiety caused by the conflict between society (mediated through the superego) and the id impulses, social structures might seem to play a major role. Admittedly, not everyone falls ill; but if society ceased its demands, there would be no illness. There would not be anything else either, since in Freud's theory it is both logically and practically impossible for society to exist without demanding instinctual renunciation of its members. However, the more civilized society gets, the more stringent its demands and 'for most people there is a limit beyond which their constitution cannot comply with the demands of civilisation' (1959, p. 191). Sometimes these demands outstrip what is necessary for the level of social organization, especially when dressed in the garb of religion. At his most optimistic (in the 1927 work *The Future of an Illusion*) Freud hoped that secularization could increase health by allowing the spirit of science (sublimated sexual instincts) to become dominant:

> Think of the depressing contrast between the radiant intelligence of a healthy child and the feeble intellectual powers of the average adult. Can we be quite certain that it is not precisely religious education which bears a large share of the blame for this relative atrophy? (Freud, 1961b, p. 47)

Social structural reform could play a role, then, in increasing the social role of the intellect.

1　**Abolishing religious education**. The route to individual and social health is for people to stop denying the full extent of human helplessness and insignificance. Religious education interferes with thought and stops us doing what can be done on earth.

2　**More realistic education for children**, which must 'steer its way between the Scylla of giving the instincts free play and the Charybdis of frustrating them' (1964, p. 149). Anna Freud developed this theme, arguing that children's natural inclinations were 'out of harmony with many of the present cultural and social habits', which stopped them sleeping and eating according to their own rhythms and deprived them of comfort sucking, skin contact and parental presence. As a result, they became 'likely to develop more of the so-called "hostility toward the id", i.e. a readiness for internal conflict, which is one of the prerequisites of neurotic development' (1966b, p. 156). In the 'Little Hans' case, Freud advocated satisfying children's sexual curiosity, to allow their thinking to develop. Both he and Anna advocated psychoanalysis for teachers and educators.

3　**Build a juster, less oppressive society**. Freud recognized that class society meant that privation was unevenly distributed. None of us are allowed to make love with our mothers, to kill and eat our fathers, but some of us are allowed to eat our fill. Privation requires instinctual renunciation, yet those who are most deprived are those who have least opportunity – through education and access to cultural resources – to sublimate instinctual demands (though presumably football and motor mechanics also permit sublimation).

Envy and hostility among the 'suppressed people' are inevitable, Freud wrote, in societies where:

> the satisfaction of one portion of its participants depends upon the suppression of another, and perhaps larger, portion – and this is the case in all present-day cultures ... A civilisation which leaves so large a number

of its participants unsatisfied and drives them into revolt neither has nor deserves the prospect of a lasting existence. (Freud, 1961b, p. 191)

But Freud insisted against Marx that eliminating the special and justified hostility of the poor towards particular historical societies can never touch the ahistorical hostility that all of us, however well-heeled, have towards society as such. In general in Freud's work (and in that of Anna Freud), the role of the real, the historical, the particular is to reinforce or modify the preset internal agenda, 'the intractable nature of man'.[5]

Particular historical societies can only partially determine our psychic fate. It is true that what happens to us affects the timing and exact form of our development, the symbols we clothe it in, our chances of health and some measure of happiness. But we bring to it an inheritance that expects, looks for and creates castration threats, seductions and other such developmental markers. Historical societies can be more or less strict about sexuality and the greater the renunciation they demand the more people prove constitutionally unequal to the task of repression and fall ill. But Society as such, civilization, always makes and must make the basic demand: that the child forego fulfilment of its incestuous wishes, which is the basis of our hostility to it. The incest taboo which we all encounter inside and outside ourselves originated in an actual event: the original parricide by a group of brothers of the patriarchal father and their ambivalence and remorse. Society, eternal society, thus becomes in Freud's theory collapsed into human nature, part of our biological inheritance. Social structures play a minor if significant part.

To sum up, in Freud's view civilization is fragile. We do not lightly forfeit the happiness of complete instinctual satisfaction. We retain impulses to aggression which no reforms can eliminate. These threaten to disintegrate the fabric of society and reduce it to 'primary mutual hostility' (1961c, p. 112). Rebellious feelings and actions are sometimes against specific injustices and thus may lead to reforms which increase human happiness within the framework of civilization. But such demands may also spring from the remains of their original 'personality, which is still untamed by civilisation ... It does not seem as though any influence could induce a man to change his nature into a termite's' (1961c, p. 96). The 'true self' here is not the radiantly intelligent child but the anarchic id. Freud concludes: 'We may expect gradually to carry through such alterations in our civilisation as will better satisfy our needs and will escape our criticisms ... but ... there are difficulties attaching to the nature of civilisation which will not yield to any reform' (1961c, p. 115).

What sorts of society, then, does Freud's conception of psychological human nature allow? Clearly no form of democracy, no enlightened organization of production, will ever completely blunt our hostility to Society itself, which is always a large part of the anger felt by disaffected groups. Social justice, the fairer distribution of power and material advantages, could minimize this disaffection. They might make it possible for the poor countries to accept environmental controls on development and for long-oppressed groups to give up war. But most of the war and pollution we face today, according to Freud, must stem from the basic hostility to Society, the aggression and greed of the rich rather than the poor. Freud's evolutionism never had to face the idea that the orderly march of civilization had itself, through the control of nature, produced disorder and death. We know today that (whether or not Freud was right in his view of the general hostility to Society) to ensure a human social future, those most privileged on an international scale will have to reduce their use of energy and their consumption generally. For this to be possible we will indeed have need of the potentially unifying power of thought, or reason, of the drive to life. On a Freudian view this possibility is inherent in psychological human nature, but its dominance can never be assured.

Chapter 5

Melanie Klein: A social emotion

Introduction

> if Kleinian psychoanalytic theory is correct, then it must have profound
> social and political implications, because it is an account of human nature
> as fundamental and wide-ranging as the accounts with which Hobbes,
> Locke, Rousseau, Marx and Freud began. (Alford, 1989, p. 197)

As Hinshelwood says, Kleinian concepts involve 'very primitive elements of the
human mind, remote from commonsense and rather like those ungraspable particles
of subatomic physics' (1989, p. 1). Although object-relations theory in general has
spread to the US and other countries, Kleinian theory has been more limited in its
influence (mainly Britain and Argentina). It is notorious for its remoteness from the
social world, yet its concepts have tremendous resonance for ecology.

   Melanie Klein was born in Vienna in 1882, Anna Freud's compatriot and fellow-
Jew but 13 years her senior. In Budapest in 1914 she was analysed by Ferenczi,
who helped her with the depression following the birth of her third child. Ten years
later in Berlin she was again analysed, this time by Abraham, who was an important
influence on her work. She became a child analyst and developed her own play
technique, which involved interpreting the transference and unconscious wishes
from the very first session, in contrast with Anna Freud's insistence on the need
first to establish a therapeutic alliance. When Abraham died prematurely in 1925
Klein moved to London, where her theories received a warmer welcome than in
Berlin. From London, through writing and at international conferences, she conducted
a polemic with Anna Freud. This became hard to handle when in 1938 the Viennese
analysts came to London as refugees and the British Society had to contain both
groups. The antagonism was particularly sharp over questions of training, for real
theoretical differences were involved. To attempt to resolve them the Society set
up a series of seminars: the Controversial Discussions of 1943 and 1944, which
succeeded only in drawing lines of demarcation. Eventually an organizational
compromise was reached by dividing the British Society into a Kleinian group, a
Middle group and a Freudian group and giving each a share of training (Sayers,
1991, p. 243).

In terms of one line of demarcation, Melanie Klein belongs with object-relations theorists as against the 'drive theory' of both Freuds. All agree that early experience is rooted in the body. However, for Freud psychic life was a function of the relationship between somatically based drives on the one hand and the internalized representatives of society on the other. The objects which allowed gratification were almost incidental to the conflict. In contrast, Klein followed Fairbairn's view of libido as object-seeking, claiming that instincts are always relational, always directed towards and experienced in terms of objects (Fairbairn, 1952). But where Fairbairn, Guntrip and others moved away from the drive theory, Klein combined the concept of internal objects with Freud's late theory of instincts. The infant's earliest bodily sensations are experienced as internal objects, gratifying or persecuting, and this experience *is* the experience of the Life and Death instincts. The Freuds make a sharp distinction between the individual and society, between which there is inevitably struggle. Society is outside the individual, although part of it is taken in. But for Melanie Klein the conflict is not between individual (i.e. the drives) and society, but between Eros and Thanatos, Life and Death, love and hate, and this conflict is enacted both internally and externally.

There is an equally deep disagreement over the nature of thought and knowledge. Our capacities to perceive and think about social reality and to be members of society are constructed, according to Klein, and the medium of construction is unconscious phantasy. Phantasy can be more or less realistic, but it cannot be contrasted with direct, unmediated understanding as in the ego-psychological model, for no such direct understanding is possible. Phantasy is the very stuff of thought. The process through which we construct ourselves, always in relation to others, is the key to the formation and reproduction of social institutions, which do not confront the individual from elsewhere and require her to adapt to them (as in ego-psychological thinking) but are both constructed and transformed by psychological processes. Thus Kleinian thinking is at the same time the antithesis of sociology and extremely sociologically suggestive and exciting in its undermining of individual-society dualism.

The nature of phantasy was one of the main lines of demarcation in the Controversial Discussions, which were so intense that participants often ignored the air raids raging overhead (Grosskurth, 1986, p. 321). Susan Isaacs gave a paper which made it clear that for Kleinians unconscious phantasies were present from birth and involved peopling the mind with internal objects. Whereas Freudian theory had the individual develop first and then form object relations, for Klein individual development happened *through* object relations – through real interpersonal relationships as represented in phantasy and linked phantasies of relations between internal objects. 'Freud had previously described hallucinatory wish-fulfilment as the mental activity of the infant in frustration. Klein ... claimed that it was an incessant accompaniment of the child's activity at all times' (Hinshelwood, 1989, p. 36). Glover thundered that phantasy had become a 'catch-all' in which 'the distinction between reality ego-systems and phantasy systems disappears. The relations between psychical reality, reality-proving and phantasy (in the Freudian sense) are obliterated' (Glover, 1945, p. 21).

Isaacs gave details of early phantasy (Isaacs, 1952). According to Klein, hunger is experienced concretely by babies as a relationship with a persecuting object actually inside them. Being satisfied is also experienced concretely as having something good inside, so that the early experience of taking-in milk becomes one of the building blocks of emotional life. Babies are also assailed by terrifying anxiety, to which they respond by phantasies based on somatic experience. They feel themselves to be expelling not only faeces but bad objects such as, prototypically, the absent, depriving breast. In phantasy they attack these hated objects through biting them up, pissing and shitting on them. Such a complex inner life implied an ego present from birth and contradicted Freud's concept of primary narcissism. Anna Freud responded:

> According to Mrs Isaacs' descriptions, the newborn infant already in the first six months loves, hates, desires, attacks, wishes to destroy and dismember his mother . . . According to my conception of this same period, the infant is at this time exclusively concerned with his own well-being. (Quoted in Glover, 1945, p. 27)

To the ego-psychologists who made the ego central to their clinical work, it must have seemed upstart cheek as well as mysticism when Klein claimed not only that a primitive ego existed at birth, but that the Oedipus complex and the superego developed during the baby's first year (Hinshelwood, 1989, p. 134).

In classical Freudian theory the superego developed through the resolution of the Oedipus complex around the age of four. According to Anna Freud, anxiety and apparent guilt in toddlers was due to fear of the loss of parents' love and could be alleviated by loving reassurance – which would have been ineffective if the superego were already formed (Young-Bruehl, 1988, p. 177). Klein, in contrast, found children of 18 months plagued by a superego that was far harsher than their real parents (Klein, 1988d, p. 402). This harsh superego would later coexist with a more realistic internal representative of society (Klein, 1988a, p. 156). As the superego moved into the pregenital period, so did the Oedipus complex. Klein found pregenital fantasies of loving and hating mother or father, of identifying with each and of a dangerous and excluding combined parent figure, made of the parental figure locked in permanent intercourse. These revisions separated superego formation from the resolution of the Oedipus complex (abolishing the idea of girls' 'weaker' superegos) and meant that the classical anxieties of castration and penis envy lost their pivotal importance (Hinshelwood, 1989, p. 64).

These, then, are a few of the main differences between the Kleinian and Freudian positions. The task of selective exposition is even more difficult in this chapter, because Klein's theory is so complex and clinically rooted. The best approach seems to be to present it in its mature form, using my questions about psychological health and the relationship between psychic and social structures as guidelines for selection.

The baby, its inner life and the external world

Freud had initially regarded the death instinct as clinically silent, which had made it easier for the psychoanalytic community to live with this speculative theoretical development (Freud, 1955d, p. 62). Klein came to believe that the incipient ego comes face to face with the death instinct, experienced as the terrifying anxiety of an object inside which is about to destroy it (Hinshelwood, 1989, p. 159). Using the primitive defence mechanisms at its disposal – introjection, projection and splitting – the baby projects its bad feelings on to the external world. At the same time it instinctively projects its libido in search of a good, life-giving object (Segal, 1964, p. 12). So the conflict which begins intra-psychically is projected outwards, because that feels safer. The question then becomes the extent to which the external world provides suitably robust recipients for these projections.

In the beginning the bad and good objects which the baby feels it has inside are not discovered but *created*. Phantasies of the objects that would satisfy instinctual aims are innate, rather than responses to parental frustration and love (Alford, 1989, p. 81). But:

> The child's experience of the external world ... is constantly influenced by – and in turn influences – the internal world he is building up ... external and internal situations are always interdependent, since introjection and projection operate side by side from the beginning of life. (Klein, 1988f, p. 138)

Real events are important in enabling the baby to sustain the necessary split between good and bad and keep her grasp on the phantasized good object, which is under threat from her own aggression and envy. The death instinct is not easily dealt with. What has been projected outside is still feared as a persecuting object. What remains inside takes the form of aggression. The baby experiences – and *must* experience – the feeding breasts or bottle as *split*, as two distinct objects: one to be feared and hated, the other desired and loved. If this seems bizarre, remember that cognitive developmental psychology confirms that knowledge of what constitutes a whole object is developed rather than given.

Only if there is a continually present good object in the outside world can the baby keep up such defences against fragmentation. What makes Klein's theory implausible in evolutionary terms is that the chips are so stacked in favour of the death instinct. 'Klein had a tendency to see bad objects as derived from the child's own drives, and good objects as derived largely from external others' (Hughes, 1989, p. 103). When the mother goes, the child's ego becomes fragmented again. The mother is not yet experienced as a whole, but in parts such as the breast and the feeling of being held. When these go, it is felt not as absence but as the presence of a bad, persecuting object (Segal, 1964, p. 13).

The terrible strength of the death instinct means that healthy development requires a preponderance of good experiences over bad. Repeated experiences of gratification, together with the development of the baby's perceptual apparatus, allow her to come to see her mother (and gradually other people too) as a whole person rather than a collection of parts: a development known as the depressive position. Assured of the recurring presence of a good object, the baby can dare to notice that bad and good are actually one. This emergence from the paranoid schizoid stage ushers in a new set of fears that this valued whole person has been damaged by the baby's own attacks. Even though most of these phantasized attacks are not acted out in ways that the mother would notice, the baby feels guilty and frightened about their effects and wants to make reparation:

> If the baby has, in his aggressive phantasies, injured his mother by biting and tearing her up, he may soon build up phantasies that he is putting the bits together and repairing her. This, however, does not quite do away with his fears of having destroyed . . . the one whom he loves and needs most. (Klein, 1988c, p. 308)

The depressive position is usually reached at around five months. It is not so much a position as a capacity, always in danger of being temporarily lost. Post-Kleinians such as Ogden argue that there is necessarily lifelong vacillation between this 'object' position (where things are done to you) and the depressive position where the self is established as subject (Hoggett, 1992, p. 83). The anxiety the depressive position brings may be so overwhelming that (in infancy or at any time of life) the ego takes refuge in the earlier state.

The perceptual-cognitive apparatus is the means of reality testing, which plays a crucial role in Kleinian thought. It can allow realistic discrimination about objects, so that phantasy itself becomes realistic. Its maturation happens automatically, unless there is some physical impediment, but its *use* is not so automatic. At first the baby equates external and internal objects. Gradually they are distinguished, in the process of symbolization (Hinshelwood, 1989, p. 432). For this step to be taken, the real safety and benevolence of the external world has to prove stronger than the persecuting fantasies which have been projected on to it:

> If anything, the Kleinian version of the environment is of something which is safer than the infant's inner world: it possesses the ability to 'contain' the infant's destructiveness sufficiently to make it tolerable and to reduce anxiety enough to allow for greater integration. (Frosch, 1991, p. 51)

If the environment is *not* benign, or cannot be experienced as such, the infant remains stuck with its own ghosts and monsters.

So far the developmental outcome is determined by intra-psychic factors mediating the effects of the external world. But in 1957, more than 20 years after her first formulation of the depressive position, Klein described the innate urge to spoil the good: envy. Now constitution again played an important role, for the strength of envy differs markedly between individuals. Envy, like aggression, is a manifestation of the death instinct arising in the earliest months of life. It does not arise merely from frustration, nor is it only felt in relation to the 'mean and grudging breast' (Klein, 1988g, p. 183), but in relation to the good one, because the baby cannot bear not being and having all that goodness. 'The very ease with which the milk comes – though the infant feels gratified by it – also gives rise to envy because this gift seems somehow so unattainable' (ibid.). Then sadistic impulses are directed against the good object itself which, if the constitutional tendency is strong, can result in schizophrenia. Envy can actually interfere with feeding, preventing the gratifying experiences which are essential if it is to be overcome.

The concept of envy led to reinforced criticisms of Klein's theory as grimly pessimistic and as underestimating the importance of the environment (Hinshelwood, 1989, pp. 175–6). It was strongly rejected by Winnicott, Heimann and others within Klein's inner circle (Sayers, 1991, p. 255). It certainly represented a significant shift of emphasis from (always psychically mediated) external factors to the baby's constitution:

> the impact of . . . external experiences is in proportion to the constitutional strength of the innate destructive impulses . . . Many infants have not had very unfavourable experiences, and yet . . . we can see in them every sign of great anxiety for which external circumstances do not account sufficiently. (Klein, 1988g, p. 230)

In this model the external world, inter-psychic processes and constitution are all operative, but constitution is once again the leading factor, mediating the effect of external factors. Such factors as sexual abuse, bottle-feeding, a calm and happy versus a fraught mother are now of less aetiological importance in the sense that their impact on development is less predictable. Is such a striking emphasis on constitutional factors the only possible response for this tripartite model, when external circumstances do not lead to the expected outcome? Another approach would be to ask whether the external circumstances were really as favourable or unfavourable as they seemed. A devoted mother, plenty of milk and lack of punitive treatment do not preclude frightening experiences – being clumsily handled, laughed at, not really noticed, not permitted to cry and so on. Perhaps this is what Winnicott meant when he wrote to Joan Riviere:

> My trouble when I start to speak to Melanie about . . . early infancy is that I feel as if I were speaking about colour to the colour-blind. She simply says that she has not forgotten . . . the part the mother plays, but I find she has shown no evidence of understanding [it] . . . The 'good breast' is not a thing, it is a name given to a technique . . . a most delicate affair and one which can only be done well enough at the beginning if the mother is in a most curious state of sensitivity. (Quoted in Hughes, 1989, p. 174)

It was partly on this issue that Fairbairn, Winnicott, Guntrip and the rest of the 'object-relations' school diverged from Klein and moved towards the view of the environment (admittedly the micro-environment of the mother-infant dyad) as the *primary* aetiological factor in development. It crucially determined how the child's inner world was formed, since internal splitting is a defensive response to environmental failure rather than instinctual conflict. In contrast, Klein viewed the child as initially creating the features of their environment by projection.

In Klein's account, one form taken by the death instinct is particularly relevant to the question of the psychogenesis of environmental destruction. Epistemophilia – the desire to know – is itself a primitive drive, a form taken by libido. The edifice of science is rooted in (though not reducible to) early curiosity about the mother's body. But, for Klein, epistemophilia becomes closely linked to aggression stemming from the death instinct. In her clinical work with young children Klein concluded that throughout their first year, babies phantasize destroying their mothers' bodies in all sorts of horrific ways, which she termed 'sadism'. Its earliest object is the mother's body, whose contents the baby in the anal-sadistic phase wants to possess and in the oral-sadistic phase to attack (Hinshelwood, 1989, p. 50). The symbolic link with postmodern and feminist accounts of modern science and the destruction of nature is striking.

Psychic structures, social structures

How does each sort of structure contribute to the reproduction of the other sort and under what conditions can this process be interrupted or transformed? Klein herself does not consider this question, so my answers have to be derived from the developments of modern Kleinians. It is fair to say that psychic structures are the more powerful in Kleinian theory, since they are innate and do not depend on social mechanisms for their reproduction. Universal constants in psychic structure – i.e. human nature – ensure the corresponding constancy of certain elements of social life, such as gender divisions, violence and destruction.

We can see a dialectic in Kleinian theory between the psychic and the social. Although the main forms of psychic structure are universal and unchangeable, the social environment has a significant influence on whether individuals achieve the depressive position and on whether and how frequently they revert to the more dangerous defences characteristic of the paranoid-schizoid position. It is not the basic psychic structures themselves, but the relative weight of one or other element which is socially influenced. The crucial social environment here is the micro-environment of the infant's first year, when good experiences are needed to mitigate the death instinct. But, although this is not spelt out, the family environment depends to a large extent on social structure in the wider sense (and this is true for object-relations theory in general as well as for Klein). It is obviously affected by the distribution of wealth and by structural and cultural factors affecting the availability, resource and self-esteem of parents. Most simply, poverty can produce anxious mothers, hunger and the frightening experience of the mother's own fear, inimical to reality-testing. The presence or absence of the father and other adults with the resources to support the mother, the degree to which she is institutionally supported, largely depend on social structures.

Even when the depressive position is achieved in infancy, social structures continue to affect the person's mental health and thus their agency throughout the lifecycle. Reality-testing remains important in adulthood. The social environment can *either* provide the conditions for reality-testing and holding on to the depressive position, *or* it can encourage or exacerbate splitting. Some institutionalized defences against anxiety hinder reality-testing and express cultural approval of paranoid-schizoid defences. Hoggett argues that present societies make it particularly difficult to distinguish between reality and fantasy and discourage thinking. Referring to Freud's patient Schreber, whose belief that the world would end in 212 years Freud confidently diagnosed as a delusion, Hoggett asks:

> whether the fantastic reality of the late twentieth century has created within each one of us, irrespective of biographical circumstance, a place perhaps sealed or encysted, a place of catastrophe, brimful of terror and despair. Is it any longer possible to know who is more deluded than whom? (Hoggett, 1992, p. 98)

Here reality-testing has become extremely difficult for all citizens. More specifically, it may be made difficult for particular groups. Institutionalized racial discrimination often results in partially segregated housing, which inhibits reality-testing for the members of both separated ethnic groups. Racist jokes produce an ephemeral and costly defence against anxiety for the hegemonic group. But racism produces its own anxieties and dangers, since treating groups of people abusively also encourages splitting and regression on their part. So while, for Kleinians, social structures do not and cannot affect the reproduction of human psychic structures as generative mechanisms, they do affect the actual form these take and whether that is healthy or unhealthy.

For Klein, violence and hatred are with us to stay, since their roots are psychic rather than social. These profoundly anti-social emotions can be partially contained by institutionalizing and channelling them (as in the army), encouraging controlled and targeted acting out. Alternatively and more effectively, they can be understood and contained by offering harmless outlets (such as sport or creative work). But containment in the everyday sense of control and limitation is only likely to work if, in the Kleinian sense, there is a person, group or institution which can act as a *container* for the negative and frightening feelings (Hinshelwood, 1989, p. 244). At best, it may be possible to enable people to recognize, accept and control their negative emotions through therapy and other practices encouraging insight. Since the path taken by particular societies is not predetermined, Kleinian theory does not entirely reduce the social to the psychic. Societies do have histories and dynamics of their own, but these are profoundly shaped by the fact that those who make history are themselves at all times battlegrounds for the instincts of life and death.

As for the reproduction of social structures, the defences against anxiety which particular social structures sanction and make available tend in turn to reproduce that form of structure:

> Social historical forces bring out certain features in the psychological development of the individual members of the society – and they inhibit others. We can postulate that capitalist society brings out in the individual personality the potential for increased projective identification (alienation). In turn projective identification spurs on the form of capitalist society. (Hinshelwood, 1983, p. 225)

We have here a two-way relationship, comparable to the models discussed in Chapter 2, using the controversial and complex concept of projective identification. Roughly speaking, this means that someone projects a part of their personality into another person, still feeling it to be part of themselves and yet experiencing it as elsewhere: I might feel that someone else is angry when the anger (which I continue to feel even while I disown it) is actually mine. This mechanism can actually result in the other feeling the anger, but experiencing it in a rather odd way. We sometimes find ourselves feeling and behaving in unusual ways when we are with particular people, which on reflection seem to emanate from their feelings about us. Bion (1984) described 'normal' projective identification as a way of communicating a state of mind, as when the infant lets the mother know how they feel, or when as empathic adults we project a perceiving part of ourselves into another in order to have their experiences in phantasy. But when the analyst, mother or other person cannot take in the communication, when the death instinct is very strong in the projector, when the projector cannot tell the difference between self and object, projective identification may be violent and desperate (Bion, 1984, p. 106). The 'literal displacement of aspects of the personality into surrounding persons' is, Rustin claims, 'a familiar feature of both intimate and even institutional life' (1991, p. 159). In capitalist society advertising and the substitution of money for earlier forms of nurturing continually encourage us to project parts of ourselves into commodities. This, certainly, is 'normal functioning'. Just as certainly this psychic mechanism reproduces capitalist society and the environmental destruction consequent upon the imperative to growth.

Does the concept of projective identification challenge the assumption of our individual separateness, or is it itself an individualist notion? Writing from a Jungian perspective, Andrew Samuels argues that the whole 'object relations consensus' on the interplay between innate and environmental factors, fails to transcend analysis at the level of the individual. Instead, it simply talks of societies on an analogy with individual psyches, an analogy that is 'biased towards wholeness' and (though he does not spell this out) ultimately functionalist, open to the same objections as the organic analogy (Samuels, 1993, p. 274):

> Object relations theories focus on intrapsychic and interpersonal explanations for personality development and dysfunction. They tend to rule out sociopolitical or other collective aspects of psychological suffering ...
> Moreover, problems in and of the development of personality will be looked

at in relation to a normative narrative of development that is not cut off from political pressures. (Samuels, 1993, p. 276)

The collective has, in his view, been reduced to the sum of individual projections. The concept of projective identification itself assumes that people are not *already* linked. Samuels challenges 'this assumption of empty space' between people (ibid.), which 'tends to feed into an approach to politics in which the irreducibly social nature of humanity has less prominence' (1993, p. 277).

Samuels' argument needs to be taken seriously. But we could look at projective identification differently – and he himself does not want to jettison the concept. We could reverse his argument by saying that for projective identification to be possible, people must already be unconsciously connected. But certainly Samuels has a point when he suggests that Kleinian object-relations theory tends to take the individual as pregiven and as then making society through projection.

Perhaps because of the emphasis on constitutional differences and intra-psychic life as the main determinants of psychic reality, Kleinians have addressed themselves more to the question of how people make society rather than how they are made by it. Rustin, for instance, in his treatment of racism nods cursorily towards imperialism and the institutionalization of discriminatory practices and focuses on states of mind (1991, Ch. 3). With a methodologically comparable thrust, Elliott Jacques, Isabel Menzies Lyth and others at the Tavistock Institute developed a theory of social institutions as collective 'social defence systems' (Hinshelwood, 1989, p. 415). In her classic study of the nursing service in a London general hospital, Menzies-Lyth argued that the primary task of an institution (here, curing the sick) and the technological resources it can muster do no more than set limits on the possible organizational forms, which are otherwise 'determined by the psychological needs of the members' (1988, p. 50). These she takes as given.

Menzies-Lyth describes the nursing situation as evoking early phantasies of damaged or dead internal objects beyond the ego's power of repair. Ideally the organization should provide help in re-experiencing these and mastering anxiety, maintaining the distinction between objective and psychic reality. In her research, the actual help offered hindered rather than promoted insight. To minimize such feelings, nurses' work was fragmented and bureaucratized, so that they could make close relationships with patients. But this institutionalized defence also kept nurses isolated and deprived them of much personal satisfaction in their work (1988, p. 64).

How do the defensive needs of many individuals produce such a social defence system? For to say merely that 'these have been projected' offers no insight into the social mechanisms involved. Similarly, Menzies-Lyth writes almost as if 'healing the sick' were a thing in itself, which confronts individuals and organizations. But in this process there are no givens. The demands the process makes on the nurse are themselves socially constructed. It might be argued that cultural understanding of sickness and death would affect what phantasies are evoked and therefore the individual's defensive requirements, which Menzies-Lyth presents as a presocial constant. Individuals only exist in society and society only exists through individuals, as was argued in Chapter 2. The nurses do not get together and make the hospital in the light of their psychological needs, for without the already-existing hospital they would not be nurses. We can never explain institutions *ab initio* in such terms, let alone socioeconomic structures such as capitalist systems.

However, this way of thinking can contribute to our understanding of social reproduction and of the possibilities and difficulties for change. If, in a given social setting, nurses' shared situation produces similar anxieties, it may be that even if they *are* allocated one patient per nurse they will use splitting to depersonalize the situation and somehow distance themselves. The partial failure of this individual defence, with the consequent anxiety, is likely to lead to the demand for social defence; for 'efficient' measures involving more specialization, the rotation of tasks and so on, which through a process of negotiation eventually become part of the formal system of rules. These are then available to new nurses as ready-to-hand defences, which will hamstring any nurse who is able to contain her anxiety and to react creatively to the situation. As Menzies-Lyth says, if there is *not* a sufficiently good matching of individual and social defence systems, there will be some kind of breakdown of the individual's relationship to the institution (1988, p. 70). This is surely the point at which proposals for new practices may be heard and even acted on.

If this approach is right, the only possible societies are those which either provide defences against the anxieties they evoke, or which provide ways of working them through. The latter is clearly preferable because it is more stable and based on real understanding instead of displacement or self-deception. The distinction is analogous to the distinction between normal functioning and positive health and offers some explanation for the yawning gap between them. Normal functioning – including denial of danger and valuation of business as usual – constitutes a defensive system. More realistic approaches to environmental threat only have a chance of success if they can provide ways of dealing with the anxiety they evoke.

Social structures, understood in their aspect of defense systems, tend to reproduce the very anxieties they defend against. Luckily societies are not monolithic. Relatively healthy individuals may be able to challenge them and bring about change, converting a vicious spiral into a benign one. In Kleinian theory such individuals depend on two social phenomena, (1) good (or good-enough) micro-social environments in infancy and (2) relatively containing and insightful social settings in adult life. Luckily such benign resources for change can persist even in societies with many abusive and destructive elements.

What is psychological health?

Does psychological health involve an element of social criticism and political activity? Probably more than any other version of psychoanalysis, Kleinian theory suggests that mental health involves a moral and political practice. To be mentally healthy in Klein's terms implies having reached the depressive position, having achieved (though never for all time) the 'developmental task' of integration (Hinshelwood, 1989, p. 325) and having a strong sense of internal and external reality. For Money-Kyrle, who wrote about morality, health and social issues in the 1940s and 1950s, there was nothing relative about it:

> The clinical conception of normality is vague. But it certainly does not depend on adaptation to society, for if it did, some people whom every clinician would class as ill would have to be classed as normal in some societies . . . We can define a normal – that is, a healthy – mind as one that knows itself. (Money-Kyrle, 1952, p. 234)

Whereas for Freud and Anna Freud altruism was a derivative of egoism and the drives, Klein believes we are innately capable of developing the capacity of concern for others (Klein, 1988c, p. 312) and mental health involves just such a development. This concern is not aim-inhibited erotic love, but a tender, social emotion based on identification and linked to pity and longing. Reparation is not a defence mechanism, though it does reduce anxiety, because 'the acceptance of reality [is] the fundamental element of real reparation' (Segal, 1964, p. 89). It involves creativity, which is also central to Winnicott's definition of health (Winnicott, 1971, p. 65). In its compulsive forms it is a defence, but it does not then embody genuine concern for others. Reparation is the Kleinian concept that has been hailed as providing a psychological basis for our moral and political desire for justice (e.g. Rustin, 1991, Ch. 1).

Money-Kyrle described a society in which psychoanalytic insight was widespread:

> abnormal divergences from the pattern of morality will have a diminishing effect on the policy of nations. Pathological prophets will be recognised for what they are . . . wars and revolutions, which are mainly products of paranoid fanaticism, passively assisted by scomotist paralysis and cynical indifference, will become less frequent. Society will become more tranquilly creative. (1944, p. 170)

Unlike Hartmann, Money-Kyrle believes that healthy people would tend to agree politically. Their relative freedom from paranoid thinking and religious illusion would make probable a 'humanist conscience' and a dislike both of authoritarian and of callous *laissez-faire* societies.

Half a century later, Rustin similarly implies that welfare socialism is the form of organization most consonant with the depressive position and with mental health. Marxist and other revolutionary movements, with their emphasis on the objective conflict of material interests between groups, positively encourage the projection of hated aspects of the self in the form of 'class hatred'. Socialists must address themselves to questions of material deprivation, but also to the quality 'and intensi social relationships of value' (Rustin, 1991, p. 37). Just because it refuses tc the ubiquity of aggressive and destructive urges, Kleinian theory, Rustin believes, is in a strong position to understand how these can be contained and modified.

If this is true, healthy human nature is at best consonant with a humane welfare socialism. There is a question as to whether this sort of society can exist except in a parasitic relationship with an inhumane capitalism somewhere else, but let that go. A more immediate question is whether reparation is as socially effective an emotion as Rustin hopes. This question brings us back to the very dispute about phantasy and reality at issue in the Controversial Discussions.

Depressive anxiety depends on our capacity to identify with others (Klein, 1988c, p. 311) and to grieve at injuries inflicted on them. We then want to 'make it better'. The difficulty is that our judgement of what injuries have been inflicted and how they can be healed may be off-beam: psychic reality can be a poor guide to external reality. From the viewpoint of the person who feels remorse, the damage done to the internal objects must be repaired. But actions that fulfil that psychological function may be inappropriate:

> The way in which such a perspective leads to insensitivity regarding the claims of real people is suggested in Klein's discussion of how colonisers, having ruthlessly exterminated native populations, might make reparation by 'repopulating the country with people of their own nationality' . . . from a Kleinian perspective the psychological effect of an act of reparation is considerably more important than its external consequences. (Alford, 1989, p. 47; Klein, 1988c, p. 334)

If the reparative urge is genuine, the person will do their best to find out the facts and what should be done. The point is that the urge to reparation is no substitute for sociopolitical analysis, which is why Rustin adds that education in *how* to make reparation is also necessary (1991, p. 35).

Reparation is more likely to be effective in interpersonal relations between individuals, which give plenty of opportunity for feedback and reality-testing. Alford argues that it is much harder for groups to distinguish reality from unreal fantasy. I can gradually come to realize (perhaps!) that the Chinese family next door are not persecutors, but there is less chance of a similar discovery in relation to China itself because of its size and distance. Alford argues that while people in their private lives usually operate on the basis of the reparative morality described as mentally healthy by Money-Kyrle, they are enabled to be sane in private life precisely because they are not so in their membership of groups. As members of the Conservative party, as Serbs or Muslims, people define themselves as not-members of another group and use paranoid-schizoid thinking. They idealize their own group and use the other as a dustbin for ancient anxieties (Alford, 1989, p. 74).

Such paranoid-schizoid thinking unleashes primitive persecutory fears, which may then result in denial of the reality of actual danger (the mechanism which, Klein argued, made the British apparently unmoved by early German bombing) (Alford, 1989, p. 77). Or people may bring about what they fear, by acting to avert an imagined external threat – Alford cites the arms race (1989, p. 74). His description is horribly in line with the current responses to ecological threat described in Chapter 2.

Similarly, Hanna Segal describes the processes of denial and splitting in public life in an article calling on psychoanalysts to show their opposition to nuclear weapons (1987, p. 3). She describes how people 'retain intellectual knowledge of the reality, but divest it of its emotional meaning' (ibid.), a defence against anxiety that makes the situation more dangerous. 'In this not quite sane situation the lure of omnipotence is increased and so is the lure of death' (1987, p. 7). The hope for individuals is that destructive and self-destructive drives can be modified 'when the individual can get some insight into his motives and visualize the consequences' (1987, p. 4). But distinguishing fantasy from reality is much harder for groups. Alford shows convincingly how modern international politics is dominated by paranoid-schizoid thinking (1989, p. 90). But is it *inevitable* that people in large groups (such as nations) should be so much less sane and less rational than people in everyday interpersonal relationships?

Although Alford grants the existence of a few reparative groups, on the whole he believes that Kleinian thought 'tragically' implies that mental health is rarely attained by people in groups and he himself accepts this conclusion (1989, p. 84). Bion, too, like Freud, sees groups as frequently aggregates of individuals in the same state of regression who have temporarily lost sight of their individual distinctiveness (1961, p. 142). However, Work Groups, whose members have an agreed common purpose, can be an exception. Hoggett tries to 'extend Bion's tentative analysis' of these by incorporating some of his later work on the 'container-contained' relationship (1992, p. 114) but he argues that in routinized everyday life, work groups constitute a sort of pretended integration. Where such groups can act as containers to transform the experience of their individual members into something 'bearable and nourishing' (1992, p. 61), they may be analogous to the depressive position. But often social agencies offer a sort of pseudo-containment ('We want to help *you* care for your family in a way that cares for the environment too, because we understand you . . . trust us . . . buy our product'), which can only work as a defence in conjunction with an avoidance of thought.

Another aspect of psychological health, for Kleinians, is the ability to think creatively. This is highly relevant to explaining the widespread flight from knowledge about ecological destruction. Bion explored the nature of thinking and knowledge and its psychological preconditions in relation to work with psychotic patients. Thinking, according to Bion, can feel extremely dangerous. Creative thinking requires a 'falling to pieces', a temporary movement into the paranoid-schizoid position, before the new views are formed in a synthesizing move (Hinshelwood, 1989, p. 387). To know is to link. It involves an emotional experience and also the capacity for abstraction (Bion, 1962, p. 51). Its development requires a 'container' (mother, analyst, society) capable of accepting terrifying and painful thoughts. Although it was written in a clinical context, one sentence from *Learning from Experience* has tremendous resonance for denial of ecological destruction:

the patient is starved of genuine therapeutic material, namely truth, and therefore those of his impulses that are directed to survival are overworked attempting to extract cure from therapeutically poor material. (Bion, 1962, p. 101)

Isn't this what we are trying to do when we glean comfort from the false reparative strategies of 'environmental management' and the 'caring' advertisements for green consumerism? For the protective shell of familiar ideas itself acts as a container, 'kept in constant repair as a defensive barrier' (Bion, 1984, p. 150). Bion remarks that 'truth seems to be essential for psychic health' (1962, p. 56). He means here not just to be told the truth, but to be able to take it in as knowledge.

Conclusion

Whether or not we accept Kleinian accounts of psychological development, the power and resonance of this conceptual vocabulary is incontestable. It provides several possible account of the phantastic origin of human attacks on our mother earth:

1   epistemophilia with its sadistic components evidenced in the notion of science as controlling nature;
2   envy and the wish to spoil the good (with the accompanying belief that there is an unlimited supply); and
3   related aggressive greed, institutionalized and disguised in the commodity form.

It can explain the attraction of illusory light green strategies as false reparation. Lastly, there is Bion's work on thinking with its clues about the flight from ecological knowledge.

Although it does not (and could not be expected to) theorize the strategy and tactics of political change, Menzies-Lyth has usefully hinted that such change may be brought about when there is dissonance between social and individual defense systems and has suggested that enduring, constructive change needs to allow the working through of very early anxieties which have been projected on to present-day social situations. Kleinian theory also shows why processes of splitting and fragmentation familiar in the radical left are so destructive to the political goals of the organizations that indulge in them.

On several counts, though, I find Kleinian theory unsatisfactory as a guide to human political possibilities. First, her account of gender remains puzzling, since on the one hand gender identity is seen as an achievement (in view of the fluidity of fantasy) but on the other hand gender is naturalized. We can rule out, from a Kleinian viewpoint, feminist Utopias which abolish sexual difference and the sexual division of labour or make sexual orientation a matter of taste. Sexual difference plays a minor role in Klein's theory, for it does not affect the nature of early anxieties and defences. In phantasy, infants – and adults – can and do occupy every possible position and have every possible sexual aim in relation to their objects. However, both boys and girls are understood as having innate knowledge – a sort of readiness and expectation rather than conceptual knowledge – of both vagina and penis. This makes the development of heterosexuality a matter of reality-testing, of phantasies coming into line with the external reality of the body. Penis envy is a secondary phenomenon. The girl envies the penis because it (along with father) are felt to be appendages of the mother (Klein, 1988f, p. 200), or she idealizes it in disillusion with the breast-mother. The nuclear family is implicitly understood as the natural container for heterosexual relations. Contempt for women and hostility towards them is explained entirely in terms of early vicissitudes, of which social structure is simply the expression. Similarly, in a book written long before Mrs Thatcher's premiership, Winnicott attributes male political domination to the inability on the part of both women and men to tolerate powerful women, 'from a fear of domination by . . . the all-powerful woman of fantasy, to whom is owed the great debt' (Winnicott, 1971, p. 165).

Klein insists, then, on the universality of sexual difference, despite the fluidity and versatility of phantasy. The implications of this position are not altogether clear, since 'to agree that the sex-distinction is ineliminable and important does not mean that one must acquiesce in received notions of the "masculine" and the "feminine"' (Elshtain, 1984, p. 84).

If environmentally destructive public policy, which is overwhelmingly produced by men, is an expression of aggression, is it committed (in fantasy at least) by all members of society, whether male or female? It could be the case that the aggression is constant, but the gender of the most obvious perpetrators is an artefact. Alternatively, the specific role of men in the military and in the power-structures of States, transnationals and so on, could be psychologically determined. The strategic implications would be different in these two cases. Could the social erections of the military machine and the injunctions on boy-children to compete and achieve, yield to reality-testing or (as Dinnerstein (1978) believes) to changes in family structure? Could social institutions be devised (by relatively healthy individuals) which allow us to work through our fear of the original all-powerful mother and our dependence on her, or are we condemned eternally to act out this fear in ways made increasingly dangerous by technological advance? If, as ecofeminists plausibly claim, practices resulting in environmental degradation are closely tied to the sexual division of labour and the institutions of male domination, these questions are vital.

Second, resolutely insisting on human similarities and with its tendency to reduce conscious agency to rationalization of the unconscious springs of action, Kleinian theory cannot take account of the sheer richness of difference between people. These differences, to my mind, can only be explained in terms of the social construction of the self and the construction of subjectivity as classed, gendered and so on. While I agree with Klein that the psychic structures which mediate experience are, in their broad outlines, common to all humans, I suspect that to understand agency and its potential we also have to look to the *particular* social processes through which subjectivity is formed.

Third, like both Freuds, Klein has no room for the idea of righteous anger. Anger is generally amalgamated to aggression and seen as an aspect of the death instinct, as destructive rather than creative. As a result, it becomes hard to distinguish the generally anti-social (an unhealthy position) from those who are angered by injustice and oppression.

Nevertheless, Klein gives incomparable focus to the problem facing environmentalists. Greed, denial, possessive individualism are institutionalized in our societies, but psychologically speaking they are rooted in fear. But when we tell the truth about environmental threat, ancient as well as present fears well up, encouraging paranoid splitting, denial and compulsive attempts to introject the good object (go out for a burger and chips, or a *cappuccino* and cheesecake). The invitation to avert global death by giving £10 a month to Friends of the Earth is somehow less comforting than the soft mouthful of goodness – and both are less frightening than the idea of *thinking* how effectively to reverse the trend towards social and ecological death. Organizations that understand these processes may be able to offer convincing hopes of effective reparation.

Chapter 6

Jacques Lacan: Exposing the myth of agency

Introduction

And then Lacan came up with a terrific trick. He started to free-associate while he was speaking, just as though he was listening. He was so good at faking associations . . . that the fascinated audience did not understand that it might have been poetry. (Clement, 1987, p. 18)

Lacanian theory . . . supplies the tools for an analysis of the way ideology, particularly patriarchal ideology, operates to construct the unconscious in particular ways, and it also produces an account of the aims and practices of therapy that contains a critique of its own claims to mastery. (Frosch, 1987, p. 271)

More than any other psychoanalyst Lacan aims to deconstruct the notion of the unitary subject as a myth, to put in its place an account of subjectivity which is fundamentally decentred from consciousness . . . the subversive implications of Lacan's position are evident. (Henriques *et al.*, 1984, pp. 212, 216)

Was Lacan a charlatan and clown, or a libertarian visionary? His pronouncements are superficially as distant from political struggles as those of Klein. Yet his 'return to Freud', in particular to the emphasis on the role of language in unconscious processes in *The Interpretation of Dreams*, has been understood as deeply radical. We shall see that Lacan only qualifies as 'radical' in a postmodern sense of the word, for which his significant contribution is his anti-humanism. For him there is no pre-existing self or ego. The subject is constructed within language (i.e. discourse). It is multiple and only tenuously held together. Our wholeness and our agency are simply stories we tell ourselves. Philosophically, then, Lacan is indeed radical: he not only goes to the roots, he digs them up. His undermining of the subject as originator of action was drawn upon by Althusser in his own anti-human

(Althusser, 1971). Lacan debunks consciousness as firmly as any behaviourist and definitely rejects biologism. But his notion of the unconscious, I shall show below, has nothing to do with social experiences. It follows that no amount of reform of social relations can improve the psyche, mend its splits or meet its desires. Lacanian theory is certainly *stylistically* subversive, patchy and pretentious yet rich, challenging and resonant. But his lack of interest in the meeting of needs in the material world and his ambiguity about the status of the real, mean that politically speaking Lacan's position amounts to no more than a provocative anarchistic conservatism.

Lacan was born in 1901 in Paris. He was educated in a Jesuitical tradition and into an hegemonic colonialist culture: a background very different from those of Anna Freud and Melanie Klein. Like Freud, but unlike Anna Freud and Klein, Lacan was a doctor, which has a certain irony in view of his later repudiation of the aim of cure. His psychiatric training had less influence on his psychoanalysis than the ideas of surrealism and phenomenology and Kojeve's lectures on Hegel.

Although Lacan presented the paper on the mirror stage (Lacan, 1977a) (later to become famous) to the International Psychoanalytical Congress in 1936, it was not until after the Second World War that he began to be well known (Lacan, 1977b). His seminars at St Anne's hospital gradually attracted larger and larger numbers, including Althusser, Levi Strauss, Merleau Ponty and other well-known French intellectuals. As dissension grew within French and international psychoanalytic circles over Lacan's practice of the 'short session', his theoretical developments and bid for independence became part of French intellectual reconstruction, rejecting the values and authority of the new American occupiers as well as the old German ones (Turkle, 1979, p. 61).

Lacan's groups, first the 'Société Française de Psychoanalyse' and, after 1964, the 'Ecole Française de Paris', were excluded from the International Society. The rows and splits only increased Lacan's fame, so by the 1970s his seminars had become a fashionable cultural event attended by about a thousand people. Most of them can have understood little, for the seminars were addressed to analysts and students of psychoanalysis and were part of their formal training. Lacan also had a research aim of a kind. For him the proliferation of psychoanalysis should permit the replicability of analytic experience and thence the establishment of psychoanalysis as a science (Roustang, 1990, p. 11). He increasingly moved away from therapeutic aims. He referred to the 'analysand' rather than the 'patient', not to subvert the power relation in the analytic relationship, but because he came to see the training analysis as the only *real* analysis. To be psychoanalysed no longer suggested functional inadequacy, but cultural perspicacity. By the 1970s his critics claimed that he was:

> throwing open another door, the door of social advancement for the psychoanalyst . . . The cure foots the bill for this whole business, it goes by the board, and the social project takes over. The psychoanalyst is no longer a therapist: he is a cultural agent, an intellectual in the noble sense of the word; his mission is to transform culture. (Clement, 1987, p. 86)

In this context we can understand the lack of systematic case material, the philo-sophical playfulness and literary quality of the seminars.

The events, in Paris, of May 1968 enhanced Lacan's status as a guru. Revolu-tionary students were attracted to his rejection of bourgeois values. Although struc-turalism was really antithetical to the voluntarism of the May events (Turkle, 1979, p. 71), these upsurges 'translated existential Marxist ideas into a kind of social action which raised questions about the world to which psychoanalysis seemed to offer some answers' (1979, p. 47).

Many of Lacan's young supporters understood his work in quasi-Marcusean terms, looking for an escape from the alienation of conventional life in dreams of pre-Oedipal unity, which Lacan completely rejected. Nor did he in any way share their political aspirations, as is shown in a 1970 film of a lecture he gave in Bel-gium. Lacan's delivery was halting and he seemed bored. He was interrupted by a situationist who harangued him and the audience for their bourgeois complacency, ending by pouring water over the desk and Lacan himself. Lacan seemed relieved by the interruption. When the young man had been removed, he spoke animatedly of the illusory nature of all searches for a New Jerusalem and of the alienated nature of such demands for an end to social alienation.

Throughout his career, Lacan provoked splits in the analytic organizations he belonged to, between his supporters and those who wanted to retain the approval of the International Psychoanalytic Association. His insistence on using the length of the session as a therapeutic tool was anathema to the establishment, which deeply distrusted him as a training analyst. Eventually he and the rump of his associates formed the Ecole Freudienne in Paris. The Ecole offered no specific training courses and was open to all (Turkle, 1979, Chapter 4). Graduation took place through the infamous 'pass'. The analytic candidate was represented before a panel by colleagues to whom he or she had entrusted her views of the course of her analysis and the reasons for her decision: the panel decided whether the analysand could become an analyst. According to Schneiderman, the colleagues did not speak for the analysand, but rather described his or her effect on them. Unsurprisingly, gossip, politics and conflicts were as rife in the Ecole Freudienne as in the organizations that preceded it. Dramatic disputes continued within the Ecole Freudienne up to its disintegration in 1980–1, just before Lacan's death:

> a large number of Parisian analysts did manage to make fools of them-
> selves ... No one could reproach analysts for having passions, but pas-
> sions by definition are suffered, not acted upon, and not spewed forth as if
> the goal of analysis were to be led around by one's passions. (Schneiderman,
> 1983, p. 46)

But what *was* the goal of analysis? Lacan's conception of it shifted consider-ably over his lifetime, but remained consistently individualist. His social thought has to be inferred from hints and throwaway remarks, or constructed on the basis of his general philosophical position.

Philosophically Lacan became increasingly opposed to psychology. He is hailed for recognizing the constructedness of the subject in language and thus providing 'a bridge between social and psychic domains' (e.g. Henriques *et al.*, 1984, p. 212), thus rejecting individual-social dualism (1984, p. 24). In fact for Lacan the individual, personal subject became increasingly uninteresting and irrelevant (Forrester, 1990, p. 118). His view of the subject as constituted by and within the Symbolic order leaves a vital question unanswered:

> in this view the subject is composed of, or exists as, a set of multiple and contradictory positionings or subjectivities. But how are such fragments held together? Are we to assume . . . that the individual subject is simply the sum total of all positions in discourses since birth? If this is the case, what accounts for the continuity of the subject, and the subjective experience of identity? (Henriques *et al.*, 1984, p. 204)

Other schools of psychoanalysis explain this common thread of subjectivity, this predictability of response, in terms of early experience – itself mediated through psychic and social structures. *This* sort of 'construction of subjectivity' is of no interest to Lacan, for whom structures organize and thus produce experience, which is thus causally impotent or redundant (Frosch, 1987, p. 193). Henriques *et al.* recognize (without its diminishing their respect for Lacan as much as I would consider appropriate) that Lacan must therefore either (1) himself illicitly assume a pregiven subject, an invisible container for these fragments, or (2) must opt for a form of discourse determinism in which people are no longer causal agents and their decisions mere epiphenomena: 'a view which leaves no room for explicating either the possibilities for change or individuals' resistances to change' (Henriques *et al.*, 1984, p. 204).

Similarly, Frosch remarks that Lacan's position threatens to slip into the 'essentialism it abhors' or 'a relentless structuralism' (1987, p. 137).

Lacan does veer between these two positions, as I shall show. In his earlier work he retains some interest in psychic processes, but increasingly the subject becomes less of a construction and more of a gap between utterances, a creature of language entirely subjected to its structure. 'The subject exists simply as the discontinuity between intention and meaning introduced by the fact that speech always occurs in relation to another speaker' (Lacan, 1977f, p. 299). It is hard to imagine the clinical implications of this position. I believe Lacan remained psychoanalytic for two reasons. First because his structuralist work was parasitic on his earlier, more psychological formulations. In his work of the 1930s and 1940s he assumes a presocial infant going through predictable developmental stages, a *psychological* conception in that the infant's understanding of its situation and its response affect the way it develops. In Seminar I, though, Lacan criticizes the psychologism of some interpretations of the mirror stage, while then and later relying on it to keep his project anchored in psychoanalysis (Roustang, 1990, p. 54). Second, Lacan's later work has its own implicit and unacknowledged psychology. Lacan reduces the subject to language with one hand and with the other silently establishes the psychological conditions necessary for us to *be* subjects constituted by language in the way he describes: in other words, our psychological human nature.

Early work: From alienation to Oedipus

Our early experience, Lacan assumed, is fragmented. Corresponding to our dependence and lack of coordination is a lack of a sense of ourselves as whole and separate. Sometime between 6 and 18 months we become aware of our reflection, both the actual mirror image and the 'self' reflected back to us from our mother. We are captivated by this image, which becomes the core of an idea of ourself as a unity. This is the birth of the ego, or *moi*. But this ego expresses not our experience, which is still uncoordinated and fragmented, but that of another: it is therefore alienated. Object-relations theory would have it that this is how we develop our intrinsically social, relating selves, but for Lacan this early sense of our separate identity is illusory because it depends on the vision of another. The child is situated only in 'physical, psychical, familial space', not in 'the larger linguistic and economic community . . . while the child remains bound to the other as its *double*, it cannot participate in society or symbolic exchange with others' (Grosz, 1990, p. 50). In the adult, too, in Lacan's conception, the ego is not the self but the site of conventional, other-given notions of the self, a fantasy of the self. It thus belongs to the order of fantasy, which Lacan terms the Imaginary.

The child at the mirror stage has, or is, a borrowed, reflected, alienated self. The very idea of alienation suggests a contrast with possible wholeness or authenticity – yet there are no such possibilities.[6] As the child becomes a language speaker, learns its name and sex, its relationship to others and its place in the world, it enters the Symbolic order, which is to say human society, as a 'speaking subject'. The Imaginary does not thereby lose its force. At the mirror stage the child is split between her fragmentary lived experience and the illusory unity of the *moi*. At the Oedipal stage she is further divided between the persisting *moi*, precipitate of her identifications with others, and her new Language-given subjectivity as a named being constituted by the web of symbolic relations (Lee, 1990, p. 65). This self too is shifting, its unity tenuous and language-dependent.

Human life begins, for Lacan, at the Oedipal moment, which is that of becoming a language speaker. This is no empirical thesis about an association between two developmental stages, as when followers of Steiner assert that children are ready to learn to read when they shed their milk teeth. In Lacan's Oedipal drama, Language (which is to say, society) is in the place of the father. Even if there is no real father, its third presence always intrudes into the mother-child couple. If there *is* a real father, he is 'always more or less inadequate to the symbolic relation . . . It is in the *name of the father* that we must recognise the support of the symbolic function which, from the dawn of history, has identified his person with the figure of the law' (Lacan, 1977c, p. 67). The Oedipus complex is not primarily a personal conflict with instinctual forces and it was only in his early work that Lacan focused on the aetiological significance in the individual case of real relations with the actual father. Oedipus is the general process of taking on a sociolinguistic identity, becoming a speaking subject with a name which situates them in a network of kin (Lacan, 1977c, p. 66). It has even been said that for Lacan, 'successful negotiation of the Oedipus conflict is quite literally a matter of learning to speak properly' (Lee, 1990, p. 64). In learning that he is a son, that his mother is his mother and his father his father, the child simultaneously learns the prohibition against incest (Felman, 1987, p. 104).

Freud used 'society' in two senses: the timeless (which I render with an initial capital) and the particular-historical. Lacan has two equivalent senses of 'language': the timeless Language and language as spoken in a particular time and place. Like Freud's, this silent distinction can blur his aetiological accounts. In what sense does Language have power over psychic development? Had it been in the sense of a particular language, a particular kinship system, we could have asked whether the Oedipus complex is universal. When discussing symbolization Lacan is certainly talking about particular languages, but the general 'Law of the Father' cuts across these, giving causal weight to Language in the timeless sense. In this case the question makes no sense (Safouan, 1981). Kinship relations are privileged, they are part of the foundation, part of Language. Even though the forms they take vary, their elementary structures are universal:

> the life of the natural groups that constitute the community is subjected
> to the rules of matrimonial alliance governing the exchange of women . . .
> The primoridal Law is therefore that which in regulating marriage ties
> superimposes the kingdom of culture on that of a nature abandoned to the
> law of mating. (Lacan, 1977c, pp. 65–6)

Lacan shows himself a very follower of Rousseau, a believer in original biological anarchy. The primordial Law, the achievement which makes us human, applies as inexorably to modern societies as to any other: 'it is perhaps only our unconscious-ness of their permanence that allows us to believe in the freedom of choice in the so-called complex structures of marriage ties under whose law we live' (ibid.). This insistence already offers a partial answer to the question: 'What is the relationship between psychic structures and social structures?' For Lacan, *historical* structures (as opposed to timeless 'elementary' ones) clearly have even less causal power than they have for Freud.

Penis and phallus

In Freud's work phylogenesis often plays the role of a *deus ex machina*, while in Lacan our linguistic inheritance plays the same role. When developmentally crucial but contingent happenings (such as castration threats) failed to occur, Freud would invoke our phylogenetic inheritance as a source of constancy, so that mere hints of castration were enough to begin the resolution of the Oedipus complex. Freud certainly believed himself to be talking about the real penis here and human subjects' inevitable non-constructed response to its possession or non-possession. For him its timeless superiority over the clitoris-vagina was evident. In fact, believing himself to be talking about the real penis, Freud was talking about a cultural fantasy of the penis in which he was so deeply implicated that its fantastic status was invisible to him.

Lacan appears to avoid such criticisms by talking about the phallus. There can be no organ superiority in the real. Real things are the way they are and such moral terms have no purchase. It is we humans, in the Symbolic register, who create and feel lack. The phallus represents both that lack and what we feel would fill it. It is a social dream of the penis: a collective fantasy of power and completeness illusorily attached to that little bit of mobile flesh. 'The phallus is not the penis, the biological emblem of the male, but a representation of the penis in which it is portrayed as the originator and possessor of a power which in fact is found outside the self, in patriarchal discourse' (Frosch, 1987, p. 197). Similarly, Lacan's idea of castration is a long way from the threat of the scissors. The 'Law of the Father' – the prohibition against incest – is the condition of membership of the human sociolinguistic order (Laplanche and Pontalis, 1985, p. 59). The threat of castration can be understood as the threat of exclusion from that order – as indeed women, the already-castrated, really are debarred from full subjectivity. But Lacan goes further. Submission to the law itself *involves* castration, in the sense of acceptance of subjection, of incompleteness. Women's consolation must be that men have to accept *phallic* castration in order to be allowed the brief measure of power that accompanies the fleshly penis.

In Lacan's system the phallus is a basic term, sometimes described as a signifier without any signified and sometimes as signifying all other signifiers, i.e. Language itself (Lacan, 1977e, p. 285). These cryptic phrases mean the same thing. For Saussure signs were the unity of the signified (the concept) and the signifier (the term) (Lemaire, 1979, p. 13). Lacan agrees with Saussure that the signifier does not stand for an extra-discursive referent. But he goes further: it does not stand for a concept either. Its meaning is given by its place in the whole network, by its difference from those signifiers that can sometimes take its place. As a signifier the phallus is unique. Our entire symbolic world is organized around the division into two sexes, which is not based on genital difference but on the attribution of a different relationship to the phallus. The phallus is unconscious, so it serves as signifier for all our substitute objects of desire, for the desire-of/for-the-mother, the breast, fast cars, money – whatever. Many things stand for it, but it stands for nothing. In this sense it has no signified. It stands for nothing in a different sense, too, because it is both fullness – a dream of completion – and absence, lack. Because no signifiers can substitute for it, it is given its meaning by the entire linguistic system: it signifies all other signifiers. This is true for all signifiers but particularly for the phallus, which is *the* unconscious signifier, the primally repressed, which does not slip and slide its meaning as less highly charged signifiers do. It lends some of its relative immobility to the whole system (Elliott, 1992, p. 136).

Thus Lacan tries to render the phallus gender-neutral, emphasizing that while half the population sport penes, *no one* can have the phallic attributes mistakenly believed to result from penis-possession (Bowie, 1991, p. 129). Some feminists are convinced (Mitchell, 1975; Mitchell and Rose, 1982) but others find it ludicrous (e.g. Gallop, 1982). The relationship of the phallus to the organ it elevates and symbolizes is not a contingent one. Why has this dream of wholeness and power – the phallus – been associated with the humble penis? Well, Lacan says, human symbol-users chose it 'because it is the most tangible element in the real of sexual copulation . . . by virtue of its turgidity, it is the image of the vital flow as it is transmitted in generation' (1977d, p. 287).

Such a naïve empiricist reiteration of the organic characteristics of the penis diverges dramatically from Lacan's usual anti-biologism. For Freud, the little boy really does want to stick his little willy into his mother's great vagina and really is scared his dad will cut it off. In contrast, the *desir de la mère* (desire for the mother/mother's desire) in Lacan's work is sexual only in a derivative, ethereal way. He tells us most implausibly that according to Freud the genital drive is formed in the 'field of culture', 'subjected to the circulation of the Oedipus complex, to the elementary and other structures of kinship' (Lacan, 1979, p. 189). Of all the drives this one is, for Lacan, most firmly detached from the body. Roustang concludes in exasperation: 'Lacan finds it absolutely essential to retain nothing of sexuality apart from lures, gaps, lack and therefore death' (1990, p. 85). Sexuality is not the product of our embodied nature, but of Language (Rose, 1982, pp. 34–5).

In Lacan the drives are constituted linguistically. Infants do go through developmental stages in which the mouth and anus play central roles, but the erogenous nature of these zones and their psychological significance are constructed retrospectively, through Language. Although the drives, carriers of desire, are post-Oedipal phenomena of the Symbolic, they are mysteriously rooted in the body. 'We see Lacan's insistence on grounding the concept of the drive in the register of the real, even if virtually all the drive's manifestations are determined by the signifying chains of the Symbolic' (Lee, 1990, p. 156).

In the 1960s Lacan discovered the *objets petit a* ('a' stands for 'autre', other, and is lower case to distinguish it from the Other of language and the unconscious). The strange list includes the breast, the penis, the gaze, urine, faeces and other products or parts of the body where something goes in or out, through a rim, through the orifices which Lacan likens to the gaps in speech where the unconscious lurks (Lacan, 1979, p. 181). Each implies a possible activity in relation to another, each represents something that was once lost. They become objects of drives, modes of the expression of desire, only as a result of the Oedipus complex and the child's acceptance of phallic loss, latecomer in the tragic series that besets him. Instinct in the animal sense seeks and finds satisfaction. The drives are psychical, language-based. They can be satisfied by a trick (sublimation) but, however satisfied, they remain insatiable.

The penis is one of the *objets a*. Why then should it be transcended into the phallus and acquire such a different status from the others? When Lacan seeks refuge in its physical characteristics to explain its privileged status, we can only conclude that for him, as for Freud, penile superiority is self-evident. He too is caught in the fantasy of our culture; unlike Freud he recognizes it as a fantasy, but claims that it is necessarily and invariably produced by human language and culture. Wherever there is speech, the penis is better. Although our dreams cannot come true, we are doomed to dream of the penis for ever: 'vulva, womb, breasts, milk and menstrual flow have, and need to have, no independent symbolic tone. They say again, in their richly circumstantial dialect, what the phallus has already said. Lacan's re-endorsement of Freud's phallocentrism is forthright' (Bowie, 1991, p. 129).

Desire: A human natural capacity

Before speech there are needs, at the level of the body; needs which can be met. Once these are expressed in speech, something is added: a further, unexpressed and inexpressible *demand* for love, for affirmation, which cannot be satisfied by any actual love. 'Words come to "stand in" for the loss of imaginary desires and loves, as the small child seeks to overcome "lack" through symbolic expression' (Elliott, 1992, p. 132). Yet this is loss as well as gain: the child moves from 'the full, imagined plenitude of the mirror phase' into that 'emptiness which is constituted by the crippling "otherness" of language' (1992, p. 135). The child thus looks to the other (the mother) for recognition and identity. This demand, as Lacan calls it in contradistinction to need, is the desire for the mother, the desire to be given this completeness by her and simultaneously the desire to be the object of her desire (the phallus). In this process the child discovers the mother's own radical incompleteness. She does not have the phallus and not only in the sense in which no one, including the father, can have it. She, as a woman, is *defined by language* as not having it, whereas men are misleadingly defined as potentially phallic. The child's desire and the corresponding lack are repressed even before consciously experienced, in what Lacan calls 'primal repression'. The phallus, which represents both the lack and what would fill it, emerges as a powerful unconscious signifier.

The speaking child has to take up a position in the human community and there is only one position they can take up – the one defined by the kinship terms whose timeless elementary forms rest on the exchange of women by men. In taking up the name prepared for it, the child accepts a position either of illusory possession or of permanent non-possession of the phallus. The 'Name of the Father', i.e. the patriarchal order in relation to which the child defines itself, becomes a metaphor for the desire of and for the mother and for the phallus. Desire itself does not go away, for we continually yearn to fill the gap we have forgotten. In so far as it propels us towards each other, it is a social impulse. But in so far as it also means that our attraction results from misrecognition, from the search for the absent phallus, it is continually doomed to disappointment and offers no foundation for an accurate perception of reality.

Lacan's concept of desire is an amalgam of phenomenology and Freud. His fundamental axiom is that 'the first object of desire is to be recognised by the other' and for that reason 'man's desire finds its meaning in the desire of the other' (1977c, p. 58). In a sense this merely expresses the 'necessarily intersubjective character of all human cognitive, affective and moral states' (Forrester, 1990, p. 138), yet it also has an unadmitted psychological, human, natural dimension. Although Lacan describes demand as an effect of speech and desire as coming from the gap between need and demand (Lacan, 1977d, p. 263), we must assume that in some inchoate prelinguistic sense this longing for recognition predates entry into the Symbolic. After all, it is the analogue of the boy's incestuous feelings towards his mother, which in Freud's schema precedes and gives meaning to the threat of castration.

In Lacan the whole Oedipal drama, its inception and its resolution, is a function of the acquisition of language. Desire emerges, giving retrospective forbidden meaning to pre-Oedipal strivings, and is repressed in the same movement. Lacan's focus on language makes this momentous change seem non-psychological, an effect of an external structure rather than of human nature. But since desire is a constant, not an effect of any particular language but of Language itself, a capacity to desire must be part of human nature. Similarly if Language is a human creation, its unvarying characteristics must be attributed to those psychological and biological capacities of human beings which allow them to create and use it. Throughout his work Lacan attributes powers and tendencies to Language, which are actually capacities and tendencies of human beings as *language users*: in other words aspects of psychological human nature.[7]

What is psychological health?

Cure? That's a dirty word – it belongs to a society they don't want to have a place in, they say; to a world in which they want to be marginal, they say; to a system they are trying to undermine . . . 'Cure' – the word repels them . . . Curing is for psychiatrists, for psychologists, for doctors, not for them, no thanks. (Clement, 1987, p. 10)

The image of the psychoanalyst that Lacan embodied . . . was that of a disciplined madness, divine but controlled lunacy . . . Lacan was so far from any idea of a responsible, respectable pillar of the community that people could see that he desired and . . . acted according to his desire. (Schneiderman, 1983, p. 111)

In his early work Lacan saw cure as a bonus. Later he rejected even the attenuated medical model of other schools of psychoanalysis. Preoccupied with the human tragedy of subjection to a castrating and castrated linguistic order, he was particularly impatient with the 'banal' ideas of health flaunted by ego psychology, suspecting that the required 'adjustment' was to the ego of the analyst. 'There is no reason that we should make ourselves the guarantors of the bourgeois dream' (Lacan, 1988a, p. 18). For Lacan the idea of rational social action is a nonsense, not a goal of therapy. He rejects the concept of agency along with the rest of Western humanism, ripped to shreds by Freud's decentring of the subject.

Lacan insists that the ego is not equivalent to the conscious subject, the I. Freud started off equating the ego and consciousness, but 'the more [his] work progressed, the less easy he finds it to locate consciousness, and he has to admit that it is in the end unlocalisable' (Lacan, 1988b, p. 8). The topography of 1920 was introduced, according to Lacan, not in a retreat from the radical consequences of decentring the subject, but in order to maintain that principle (1988b, p. 11). Now that Freud no longer identified the ego with consciousness, it could not be equated with the subject. The power of the other two agencies in the divided mind was brought out even more strongly. This was not understood: 'there was a general rush, exactly like kids getting out of school – *ah! Our nice little ego is back again! . . .* there was satisfaction in being again able to believe the ego to be central' (Lacan, 1988b, p. 11).

Far from being the potential seat of rational agency, the ego (the *moi*) is for Lacan the origin of the resistances and the source of compulsive obscurity (Lacan, 1977b, p. 15). As far back as 1948 Lacan rejected Freud's description of the ego as in touch with reality. He castigated Freud's 'surprising' failure to recognize 'everything that the ego neglects, scomotises, misconstrues in the sensations that make it react to reality, everything it ignores, exhausts, and binds in the significations it receives from language' (Lacan, 1977b, p. 22). Where Anna Freud stresses that the ego is the only agency the analyst can speak to and observe, Lacan observes triumphantly that her book itself shows that the ego 'is structured exactly like a symptom. At the heart of the subject, it is only a privileged symptom, the human symptom *par excellence*, the mental illness of man' (1988a, p. 16). (He adds disingenuously that this is a dazzling insight.) In other words, our belief in our identity is rooted in fantasy, not reality, since it ignores our internal splits and our subjection to language. We believe in ourselves, which Lacan calls 'a common enough madness' (1988b, p. 12), not recognizing that we are constructed in the image of others and in thrall to the Other, the unconscious/Language (Elliott, 1992, p. 138). Like other symptoms, the ego is a compromise formation that rations and diverts desire.

We have seen that Lacan disinguishes the *moi*, the ego, from the *je*, the self the child acquires when it becomes an acculturated, gendered being. One aim of analysis was to show the subject the illusory nature of his/her identity, undermining that very certainty which is often taken as the mark of sanity. The analysand's speech was the mouthings of the ego, that alienated precipitate of others. The aim was to replace it with 'full speech', the voice of the *je*, which alone could tell the subject's story in a way that made sense of the present by including material from the unconscious 'censored chapters' (Lacan, 1977c, p. 88). This could happen through

?

an analytic dialogue, in which the analyst makes sense of the chain of associations by punctuating them (for instance, by the notorious 'short sessions'). He may
sparingly interpret, but the aim of interpretation is not so much to reach insight
as to prevent pseudo-insight through complacent objectifying self-description ('I
am an obsessional neurotic'): a new *moi*. Lacan considered an analysis a failure if
it ended with the analysand identifying with the analyst.

When the subject speaks fully he becomes the hero of his own narration,
emerging 'from the protracted sleep of analysis, not to luxuriate in being but to face
the real and perhaps to act according to his desire' (Schneiderman, 1983, p. 103).
The process was not so much therapeutic as ethical. To face the real included
facing death – the parallel with Freud is clear. Both Freud and Lacan put ethical
value on recognizing truth, but they have different ideas of it. For Freud, the moral
realist, mental health involved engagement on the side of reason and civilization.
For Lacan, precursor of postmodernism, it involved perceiving the relativity of
such ponderous values and preferring the honest individualism of *style*. Not only
the rigidity of recognized symptoms, but also the symptomatic rigidity of 'normality' must be replaced with fluid awareness of one's own divisions, multiplicity and
the assumption of one's desire.

Yet there is something puzzling here. All hinges on the assumption of desire,
without which (since we have ditched convention) life would have no purpose and
no style. But how can Lacan vehemently reject the illusions of the ego, yet recommend a life spent assiduously chasing illusory substitutes for the phallus? Indeed,
later Lacanian theory has a different aim, reminiscent of Freud's *Analysis Terminable and Interminable*: to recognize that the *je* too is 'castrated', permanently and
inescapably fractured and to give up all aims of unity and wholeness. The subject
is *subjected*: 'the subject is subject only from being subjected to the field of the
Other' (Lacan, 1988b, p. 188). Acceptance of subjection/castration takes different
forms for men and women. For boys and men, possession of a penis leads to
lifelong anxiety about whether it really has phallic properties and a vain search for
proof in sexual performance and in a fantasy of Woman as 'the Other', 'made to
stand for its truth' (Rose, 1982, p. 50). One of the aims of analysis for men is to
get them to accept that they cannot have the phallus.[8]

For girls and women, the desire for the unattainable phallus takes the form of
attempts to *be* it (by completing men or competing with them) or to *have* it through
sex and babies. This search is fruitless. Fulfilment or psychological health cannot
be found in sexual pleasure, in which the two people are invariably separate since
each is relating to an imaginary phallus rather than to a real human being – 'there
is no sexual relation' (Lacan *et al.*, 1982, p. 141). Yet though women are even less
likely than men to accept castration by giving up these illusions, in another way
they may have the edge on men. For if health lies anywhere, it is in facing the truth,
the real. In the 1970s, in his seminar *Encore*, Lacan talked about the *jouissance*
in the real that we all have to give up when we enter the Symbolic and begin our
lifelong quest for the Holy Phallus (Lacan *et al.*, 1982, p. 141). This is reminiscent
of Freud's description of the delight in odours that humans gave up on becoming
bipedal and assuming civilized restrictions (Freud, 1961c, p. 106). Just because of

women's double castration, Lacan suggests they may retain access to wordless, immediate experience – but since they cannot say anything about it, it remains elusive (Lacan *et al.*, 1982, p. 145; Lee, 1990, p. 184).

Psychic structures, social structures?

Lacan is often taken to be a social constructionist, who charts the construction of gendered subjectivity in particular societies. Such a view is profoundly mistaken. Just as Freud was concerned with timeless Society rather than with historical societies, Lacan is concerned with Language rather than languages, with *the* linguistic order rather than the orders associated with particular cultures. It is therefore a mistake to say, as Grosz does, that:

> Lacan's distinction between the penis and the phallus enables Freud's biologistic account of male supremacy and women's penis envy to be explained in linguistic and symbolic, and thus *historical* terms ... This had the major advantage of enabling the possibility of change to be articulated. (1990, p. 123, my emphasis)

The relationship between the social and the linguistic is obscure in Lacan's work, but it is clear that he does not attribute significant causal power to the historical. While the linguistic order may slip and slide, it is anchored by the *point de capiton* (upholstery button) of the ahistorical phallus.

Turkle similarly tries to sociologize the phallus in what is supposed to be an exposition of Lacan's position: 'the phallus serves as a distinctive feature that separates two classes of objects, men and women. In our society, these classes are not equal, and the phallus as signifier is the carrier of this information about social inequality' (Turkle, 1979, p. 75). Lacan himself does not offer much joy to such a reading:

> It should be made clear that this advocacy of man's relation to the signifier as such has nothing to do with a 'culturalist' position in the ordinary sense of the term, the position in which Karen Horney, for example, was anticipated in the dispute concerning the phallus by a position described by Freud himself as a feminist one. It is not a question of the relation between man and language as a social phenomenon, there being no question even of something resembling the ideological psychogenesis with which we are familiar. (Lacan, 1977e, p. 285)

No foothold for sociology here.

To build a social constructionist theory on Lacan's work may be a useful project,[9] but to pretend that Lacan has already theorized subjectivity in sociohistorical terms is confused and confusing. Thus Banton *et al.* hail Lacan's rejection of the idea of a rigid timeless psychological human nature (Banton *et al.*, 1985, p. 54), when this is just what Lacan upholds. The mirror stage, the axiom that the 'first object of desire is to be recognised by the other', are, I have argued, elements in a theory of psychological human nature. If Language, in all its causally relevant aspects, is an unchanging given, then it is not the constructor of an historicized human nature, but coterminous with a timeless one. The 'passion of the signifier', Lacan writes:

> becomes a new dimension of the human condition in that it is not only man who speaks, but that in man and through man it speaks (*ça parle*), that his nature is woven by effects in which is to be found the structure of language, of which he becomes the material. (1977e, p. 284)

Lacan has his own variety of foundationalism. Language becomes the foundation on which rest social forms and human yearnings and it has its own materiality: 'It is a subtle body, but body it is' (Lacan, 1977c, p. 87). But if Language in general is the foundation, the differences between languages have to be assumed and unexplained, as does the development, the diachronic succession of networks of signifiers, of any one language. We cannot turn to the social as an ordinary materialist would do to explain, for instance, the *glissage* in gendered words such as 'master' and 'mistress' and other examples beloved of feminists. To do so would reverse the relationship Lacan has claimed, in which the differences between men and women are neither anatomically determined nor socially constructed, but the result 'of the pre-existing oppositions between the clusters of signifiers in the system of language' (Lee, 1990, p. 176). Practices based on language structure cannot be invoked to explain changes in that structure.

Nor can social structures have any independent extra-discursive effect on psychological development, for Lacan's conception of society is as a symbolic rather than a material order. In the development of his work the real loses what causal power it had when, back in the 1930s, it simply meant the external world independent of human will. Lacan distinguished three registers: the Imaginary, the order of fantasy, prior to discourse; the Symbolic, the discursive order; and the real, the extra-discursive. In the postwar period the real remained the extra-discursive, but its features were not in any sense *productive* of linguistic categories. Instead, the real was now what *could not* be symbolized. It is featureless, confused; 'It is the world of words that creates the world of things – the things originally confused in the *hic et nunc* of the all in the process of coming-into-being' (Lacan, 1977c, p. 65). This is a version of linguistic idealism. In this middle period the Symbolic included the unconscious, which was 'structured like a language'. By the 1960s the real had become identified with the unconscious and the world a pale fantasy of thought. Not only the concept of the real, but also that of the unconscious had significantly altered. The real became a lack, a gap, known through the failures and ruptures of language (Roustang, 1990, p. 75), an order which could not be known, but sometimes evoked by poetic and outrageous intellectual gyration. Whatever the real meant, it did not mean social structures, which clearly lack causal power in this schema.

Another way in which Lacan has been mistakenly thought to allocate social structures a significant influence on development stems from a confusion between Language and society. Banton *et al.* describe the unconscious in Lacan's theory as 'socially formed' (1985, p. 54). Certainly Lacan believes the unconscious is formed through the acquisition of language, through the primal repression of forbidden signifiers, but it is not an effect of social structures. The unconscious is not primarily individual. Its contents are what is forbidden (by the law of the father) rather than what is painful, which itself minimizes idiosyncracy. 'The unconscious is that part of the concrete discourse, in so far as it is transindividual, that is not at the disposal of the subject' (1977c, p. 49). Sometimes Lacan does seem to suggest that we each have an unconscious mind, but he still sees it more as an absence than a presence. This is no reservoir of libido, but gaps, spaces, discontinuities and substitutions: things that cannot be said or thought.

Klein (1988b, p. 225) thought she was gaining access to Dick's unconscious when she interpreted his play with trains in terms of Dick going into his mother and the child reacted dramatically. According to Lacan she was *giving him* both language and the unconscious, in the same act. For 'the unconscious is the discourse of the other' (Lacan, 1988a, p. 85). Lacan's is not a psychological conception:

> There is nothing remotely like an unconscious in the subject [i.e. Dick]. It is Melanie Klein's discourse which brutally grafts the primary symbolisations of the Oedipal situation on to the initial ego-related inertia of the child. Melanie Klein always does that with her subjects. (ibid.)

If for Klein the subject creates the social world out of phantasy, for Lacan Language creates the subject and the social world.

My question is answered. Lacan has reproduced the Freudian conflict between biological individual and Society, but his version is like a shadow puppet-show where sexuality resides in signifiers and Society has become Language. The human tragedy is not our powerful drives, but our intrinsic desire for fullness which the otherness and insubstantiality of Language must always frustrate. *This* human tragedy is actually less easy to modify than Freud's. Education, psychoanalysed teachers, good mothers, kind fathers and the enlightenment of children are all beside the point. As for sexual difference and the psychological distress associated with it, this is not the effect of social structure in any meaningful sense. Feminists like Gallop claim we can accept the 'Law of the Dead Father' while struggling against the 'rule of the actual living male' (Gallop, 1982, p. 14), but for Lacan the Law of the Father is the law of culture itself.

Political possibilities: Lacan and others

Lacan was obviously aware of the differences between societies, but he did not see them as making much of a difference. Both authoritarian and libertarian, he advocated no particular politics. He never encouraged identification with humankind, an idea which he saw as repressing subjectivity and personal style (Schneiderman, 1983, p. 112). He rejected ego psychology's aim (common to most psychotherapy) of putting the ego at the helm: in his view this version of sanity inevitably led to paranoia. Schneiderman claims that Lacan's apolitical stance was a political one in disguise. Lacan refused 'to call on the consciousness that had produced the Holocaust and ask it to minister to the survivors. He would not require consciousnessness to show itself strong enough to integrate the madness it had itself unleashed' (Schneiderman, 1983, p. 177). If Schneiderman is right, Lacan's mistrust of the ego (of which the conscious mind is part) made his pessimism about human beings' capacities to build good societies even more profound than Freud's.

We only exist as subjects in so far as we are language speakers. We look to the Other (to Language and the social relations it governs) for our identity, our wholeness, but it too lets us down. For language is not solid and cannot lend any solidity to our identity. It cannot put us in touch with any extra-discursive essences, for it is composed entirely of signifiers. There is no meta-language. Thus Lacan concludes that both subject and Other are permanently castrated. To translate this odd statement into the more familiar language of my questions: human nature entails that we will always look for final recognition and affirmation of our identity, which we can never get. This will be true in all societies, so the differences between them are insignificant and the search for the good society an illusion. The very question of what actions should be taken to avert environmental threat contains this illusion, for it appeals to the Other, implying the possibility of guaranteed knowledge of an extra-discursive realm. Even if this question were provisionally answered, we are probably incapable of social engineering to satisfy our material needs, because we are in no sense rational agents. We do not know ourselves: we are fragmented and volatile: desire, which is inherently incapable of being satisfied, will prevent our meeting humankind's physical needs. The Messianic idea put forward in the thesis of sociopolitical change to save humankind is just another Imaginary dream of the phallus, an impossible dream of wholeness and restoration.

This suggests that politically speaking Lacan was far more pessimistic than most other psychoanalytic thinkers. For them, the key feature of psychoanalytic thought is its emphasis on the aetiological role of unconscious processes. The unconscious acts both as a resource of energy and creativity, constitutive of society, and also as a constant internal saboteur that undermines its most valuable creation, the rational thinking moral subject. It diverts human action into the repetitive compulsions emanating from destructive aspects of the drives. For Lacan, there is no rational thinking moral subject.

Chapter 7

Humanistic psychology: Saved by synergy

Introduction

We turn now to humanistic psychology, which embraces independence of social conventions as part of its notion of mental health. Humanistic psychology is as diverse as psychoanalysis. It is united only by the principle that the true, original self is naturally social and cooperative and that both inner conflict and social evil are environmentally produced. There is not such a gulf between psychoanalysis and humanistic psychology as my selection of theorists might suggest. Ego-psychology's 'conflict-free zone' of the ego begins to bridge the gap. Horney, Fromm, Sullivan and the 'culture school' identify patterns of defence as typical of entire societies and as products of their culture (e.g. Sullivan, 1964, p. 70). Reich (1968) believes that genitally healthy people, capable of surrendering themselves in genuine orgasm, would be socially cooperative, non-authoritarian and self-regulating. The mismatch between society and our real, genital selves is merely 'the artifact of a sex-negating culture' (Reich, 1968, p. 232). And as we have seen, for object-relations theorists such as Fairbairn, Guntrip, Winnicott, Kohut and Kernberg the individual's internal world is significantly affected by the environment, as 'formed in the cataclysmic encounters of childhood and perpetuated in the depths of the unconscious' (Frosch, 1987, p. 94). Social relations are key to the construction of the self. Aggression tends to be reactive and the drives operate in the service of a relationship-seeking ego. If the social environment allows the child's needs to be met (including its need for love), theoretically internal splitting can be avoided.

The theories so briefly mentioned here form a philosophical bridge between psychoanalytic and humanistic theories. For this very reason, the conflicting principles involved in this area are more clearly extracted from the theories on either side of the stream. From the psychoanalytic side, object-relations theories are frequently accused of having gone over to humanism, to the territory of the 'true self' and the 'whole ego' (Frosch, 1987, p. 107). We have seen how contemptuous Lacan was of ego-psychology, of its faith in the ego's susceptibility to reason. For him, too, American ego-psychology and humanistic psychology were both revisionist idiocies which elevated that illusion: the conscious self as ration order to assess these criticisms we must now cross the water to the territory of the 'human potential movement'.

The gulf between humanistic psychology and psychoanalysis is more a matter of culture and history than of theory. If some psychoanalytic strands share 'typical' features of humanistic psychology, the European and psychoanalytic sources of humanistic psychology can often still be traced. Transactional analysis (TA), for example, shows none of the humanistic concern with 'positive health'. It shows its origins in ego-psychology in its view of the child's 'life position' (view of itself in relation to others) and 'script' (compulsive dramatization of that view) as taken up in response to the drama of early experience in the family, including the Oedipal triangle (Berne, 1975, p. 125). Harris, TA's founder, even shared Freud's view that Society in general, with its necessary and frustrating demands, rather than oppressive features of particular societies, creates the typical and distressing 'child-hood situation' of 'I'm not OK' (Harris, 1973, p. 42). What puts ego-psychology on one side of the fence and classical TA on the other is culture and history rather than theory. Like psychoanalysis, TA sees no intrinsic value in the expression of feelings. These are often 'rackets' (i.e. inauthentic). Even authentic feelings, the province of the 'Natural Child' ego state, should only be released when the respons-ible, calculating Adult part of the self decides this is appropriate (Harris, 1973, p. 32). It offers no 'peak experiences', prompting one psychoanalytic commentator to complain: 'TA appeals precisely by staying away from the extremes of experi-ence, and so unifying people, through its groups, with the compact majority in the middle' (Kovel, 1977, p. 176).

We can ignore the accusation of conformism, which does not apply to most recent versions of TA. Nevertheless, Kovel does point to one of the humanistic aspects of TA: do-it-yourself. Humanistic psychology can be heavy and technical to read, but it never approaches the difficulty (or arguably the subtlety) of psycho-analytic theorizing. The therapist may be a professional, but not to the same extent a member of an esoteric group whose knowledge and authority is vital to the heal-ing process. The client is a growth-seeking consumer, rather than someone in the sick role; and the professional is educator as well as therapist. Although humanistic psychology does claim success with deeply distressed people, the doctor-patient model is no more than a temporary expedient to be transcended as soon as possible. In general the transference is discouraged, although some forms of humanistic psychotherapy do work with it. Humanistic psychology offers directions for living, where psychoanalysis aims to effect its psychic restructuring largely in the analytic hour, assuming that after a while the analysand will spontaneously act differently.[10]

Behavioural change is often among its goals, but humanistic psychology does not share the unreflective conformism of behaviourism. Like classical psychoana-lysis, it rejects adjustment as a goal and argues for the objectivity of criteria for health. If its goal is to change behaviour, this is only in the service of its ideals of positive health. It does not endorse the behaviourist view of the mind as a 'black box'; nor reduce action to behviour. Behavioural change is partly valued as a way of accessing and affecting feelings. For humanistic psychology, people act in cer-tain ways because they expect to achieve a certain valued end (which may not be anything they have experienced before) and because that course of action has a certain meaning for them. However, if convinced, intellectually and experientially, that this expected end cannot be reached this way, or that the attributed meaning is inappropriate, people can decide to do otherwise. No specific reinforcement is necessary, as it is in behaviourist models.

In this area of decision and redecision humanistic psychology has an unlikely family tie with Jacques Lacan in the shape of common ancestors – existentialism and phenomenology. This heritage is mediated by existentialist psychotherapy, which sees both behaviourism and psychoanalysis as mechanical: both offer casual explanations of people's development and actions. It draws on Husserl's phenomenology, advocating the description and study of the actual data of experience, free from abstraction and presupposition (a view which in these post-Kuhnian days seems astonishingly naïve). Maslow speaks of 'innocent cognition' (1973, p. 261) and he and others cite Eastern philosophy in their advocacy of the 'here and now'. Phenomenology is anti-naturalistic: it claims that human experience can only be studied on its own terms, from within; that such study must be interpretive and hermeneutic. Experience is foundational, the only validator for phenomenological psychotherapists. To tell someone you know more about their mind than they do is seen as dangerously arrogant (Laing, 1961, p. 14), which rules out the Freudian concept of the unconscious. Despite their scruples, existential psychotherapists do seem to know all about us. They know that our pathology (our routine banality as well as our neurotic games) comes from our fear of actually experiencing the present, including our awareness of mortality. Once we gather the strength to face death and alienation, we will be freed from the false meaning convention lent us; free to choose and to create our own life's meaning.

This idea of choice is central to humanistic psychology, which offers a sort of spiritual version of the rags-to-riches myth. Real events do matter, because they produce the bad decisions that dog us and because we insist on living as if the present were the past. But we are free at any moment to redecide – freedom is at our fingertips. Amusingly, American humanistic psychology spat out part of the European legacy of existentialism:

> I don't think we need take too seriously the European existentialists' exclusive harping on dread, on anguish, on despair and the like . . . This high IQ whimpering on a cosmic scale occurs whenever an external source of values fails to work. They should have learned . . . that the loss of illusions and the discovery of identity, though painful at first, can be ultimately exhilarating and strengthening

reprimands Maslow (1968, p. 16).

As we have seen, Freud argued that the distinction between well and ill people in emotional terms was a pragmatic one, since the processes implicated in pathogenesis are the very same as those involved in normal development. Humanistic psychology has taken a further step away from the medical model. It rejects many of the diagnostic labels used in psychiatry, refusing to reify the 'diseases' they name.

Similarly it challenges psychoanalytic categories like 'narcissistic' or 'paranoid'. Humanistic practitioners are more likely to describe people in terms of their ways of responding to social situations, or in terms of the capacities they use or fail to use, so that the distinction between the well and the ill begins to look more like one between aware people with good habits and strategies and people with bad and ineffective ones. Rational-emotive therapy, for instance, on the humanistic behavioural borderline, basically teaches clients to infer their irrational beliefs from how they react in 'upsetting situations'. Ellis shows his clients, by argument, that irrational beliefs such as 'I am worthless if I make a mistake' are both wrong and depressing and trains them to substitute more rational and cheering beliefs (Ellis, 1974, Ch. 4).

In psychoanalysis the rejection of the medical model resulted in theories of human nature which extrapolate from the struggles of those who are subjectively distressed or labelled 'mentally ill', while this same rejection in humanistic psychology has resulted in its focus on the positive dimensions of health. It asks not how humans are forever limited, but of what they can be capable at their best. No wonder it is the chosen approach for the green movement. If the promise of humanistic psychology holds good, if congruence between society and its members is achievable, if rational action by individuals and collectivities can be brought about, ecologism may have a long-term and effective future.

Human nature and the real self

Abraham Maslow was a co-founder (with A. J. Sutich) of the *Journal of Humanistic Psychology* and a leading theorist of the 'third force' (the other two forces were psychoanalysis and behaviourism) ever since its emergence in the 1940s. Human beings as a species have an intrinsic nature, exemplified in individuals, but the balance of human natural capacities is not exactly the same in all individuals. All have the need for love, for instance, but not all are musically talented. Both the shared human nature and the individual forms it takes can be scientifically studied and we can 'discover what it is like (discover – not invent or construct)' (Maslow, 1968, p. 191). As for its content:

> the basic human emotions and the basic human capacities are on their face either neutral, pre-moral or positively 'good'. Destructiveness, sadism, cruelty, malice, etc. seem so far to be not intrinsic but rather . . . violent reactions against frustration of our inner needs, emotions and capacities. (Maslow, 1968, p. 3)

Rogers, founder of 'person-centred counselling' concurs:

> I find that man, like the lion, has a nature . . . whose deepest characteristics tend towards . . . cooperative relationships, whose life tends fundamentally

to move from dependence to independence; whose impulses tend naturally to harmonise into a complex and changing pattern of self-regulation
... such as to preserve and enhance himself and his species. (Rogers,
1990, p. 405)

For Perls, father of Gestalt, this inner nature is consistently stultified by social
demands. We are part of nature, but:

that our life is not consistent with the demands of society is not because
nature is at fault or we are at fault, but because society has undergone a
process that has moved it so far from healthy functioning that our needs
and the needs of society and the needs of nature do not fit together any
more ... it becomes doubtful whether a healthy and fully sane and honest
person can exist in our insane society. (Perls, F. S. 1972, p. 18)

Society was once in tune with human nature and the environment, it seems, and
could be so again.
   That human beings do indeed have a species nature is a theme of this book.
It consists, as Maslow *et al.* indicate, of certain capacities, tendencies and needs.
These can only be known through their effects, at the level of events, and such
events will be multiply determined. So far there is no disagreement with psychoanalysis. The first quotation, from Maslow, needs to be supplemented with his clear
account of where these approaches do diverge:

'Evil' behaviour has mostly referred to unwarranted hostility, cruelty,
destructiveness, 'mean' aggressiveness. To the degree that this ... is
instinctoid, mankind has one kind of future. To the extent that it is reactive
(a response to bad treatment), mankind has a very different kind of future.
(Maslow, 1968, p. 195)

In a good society, which was oriented towards meeting human needs, human
beings' true nature would emerge. Whereas for psychoanalysis (always excluding
Lacan) such a society would contain, channel and minimize destructive, anti-social
impulses and actions, for humanistic psychology a genuine parallelism between
social institutions and human nature is attainable. This is *synergy*, which rewards
cooperative impulses rather than greedy ones.
   On what grounds do Maslow *et al.* privilege our pro-social, cooperative
impulses as natural, real and authentic? For obviously humans are *capable* of
everything they do, so violence and anti-social activity must, in this sense, be
part of human nature. In any case, what constitutes anti-social activity depends on
social context, whereas our real human nature is presumably timeless. Certainly
legitimized violence might well be seen as pro-social, as necessary to child development, for example, or to the reformation or punishment of miscreants. Even
when disapproved of, it is not obvious why these traits should be seen as distorted
forms of human nature. The ethological argument which explains why the stereotyped

behaviour of a caged lion is a distortion of its real nature is hard to apply to humans, whose proper environment, society, is intrinsically variable. There are two answers to this question, one implicit and one spelt out.

The implicit answer depends on a version of Darwinism. Although we are not caged lions, since society is a human creation, there is some analogy. The societies in which we evolved are far behind us. We retain our self-healing capacities and tendency to psychological growth, a movement towards autonomy, but the societies we have since built do not provide good conditions for their use. Rogers speaks of the 'wisdom of the organism' which is hidden from our conscious mind by our defences so that 'consciously we are moving in one direction, while organismically we are moving in another' (Rogers, 1990, p. 406). The authentic and real parts of human nature are, then, our pro-social biological (genetic) inheritance, which is realized when our needs are met.

This brings us to the explicit answer, which refers us to human needs. Humans thrive when these are met, both in the process of development and in adulthood. It is therefore appropriate for us to value (and see as healthy) whatever social arrangements best meet human needs (Maslow, 1973, p. 7). This includes human capacities, such as the capacity to read or to dance: 'Capacities clamour to be used ... that is, capacities are needs, and therefore are intrinsic values as well' (Maslow, 1968, p. 152). In general, humans suffer when their needs are not met and this suffering is a *prima facie* reason for meeting them. However, various defensive processes – which are also human – slot in to mask some of this suffering, so that we can be deceived by the bonhomie of the pub, the temporary delight of the consumer's satisfied greed. Such normal addictions and distractions, as well as neurosis, other forms of 'mental illness' and 'personality disorders' are all defences developed to deal with the painful effect of unmet needs. Side by side with the tendency to growth, with the capacity to tune in to the small, quiet voice of our instinctual nature, is another, also human, tendency to go back instead of forward in search of safety. We also have the human tendency to react to frustration with anger and powerful action. This is healthy when it leads us to change the environment (Clarkson, 1989, p. 10). 'It is the act of repressing them – the setting up and maintenance of the grim clinch of the musculature – that makes these aggressions seem so wasteful, "anti-social" and intolerable' (Perls, Hefferline and Goodman, 1951, p. 149). Where psychoanalysis remains ambiguous about the extent to which we can dispense with defences, humanistic psychology is clear. They can all go and in a state of individual and social health they are not present.

There is a considerable danger of circularity here. How do we know which human traits are part of our real nature? For instance, why should lovingness, cooperativeness and clear thinking be so identified? Supposedly because they enable humans to thrive, but this is not necessarily the case. Their objects may thrive (sometimes), but those who exercise them may well be persecuted or despised. Because they lead to growth? But do they? What is growth? Because in a good society such traits would be praised and would lead to the wellbeing of those who had them? But this returns us to the question of criteria for a good society, i.e. a society in which people's needs are met, so that they are loving, cooperative and clear thinking. We *can*, as argued in Chapter 3, argue for universal criteria for individual and social health, even though these must remain schematic and contested. Such arguments will require evidence about the nature and types of human capacities, satisfactions and suffering. To suggest that only healthy aspects of human nature are 'real' aspects goes further. It should be understood, I believe, as prescriptive rather than descriptive. It encourages us to resist the idea of 'original sin' and its psychoanalytic equivalents. We are born good, before the Fall. The Fall is human, but it is not inevitable and therefore not 'real'. And however far we fall, we can reclaim our innocence and joy.

Needs and the vicissitudes of the self

It should be clear by now that humanistic psychology has deep disagreements with psychoanalysis about the nature of the self. Like Freud it sees the instinctual self as the site of individuality and the social self as the source of conformism. But for the 'third force', the instinctual self is not anti-social, but reliably constructive: while the conformity elicited by the social self can be anti-human, except in the society where our current nature originally evolved and in the future Good Society (or Societies). How does this happen? I will briefly overview the views of Rogers, Perls and Maslow.

For Rogers, 'unconditional positive regard' is a necessary condition for children to develop well and for a person of any age to draw on their capacity for self-healing. This may be likened to the 'container' of Kleinian theory or the therapeutic alliance of ego-psychology and its lay equivalents, for it does not imply collusion by therapist, parent or social authority figure – merely unconditional commitment to the person and their wellbeing. This is, indeed, an emotional need. Its satisfaction permits the person to develop and to trust their intuition, to rely on it to discover 'that course of action which would come closest to satisfying all his needs in the situation, including needs for enhancement, for affiliation with others and the like' (Rogers, 1990, p. 415). But without loving and safe relationships in which to deal with difficult happenings and feelings, the person may become unable to distinguish the present from the past, or unable to recall certain painful experiences, with the concomitant loss of some emotional and thinking capacity. In other words, they may become distressed or neurotic.

In Gestalt therapy a person who is healthy lives awarely in the present. When they notice a feeling or sensation – thirst, or the desire for companionship – this becomes a clear 'Gestalt', i.e. a figure separate from its background. They mobilize their energy to act on the environment to meet that need or want; then, basking in satisfaction, they move back into equilibrium until a new 'Gestalt' emerges. Human beings have an inherent need for wholeness (Korb, Gorrell and Van De Riet, 1989, p. 26), and when needs are unmet the unfinished business remains in mind, preventing full present-time awareness. 'The way to happiness is starting to be happy right away ... we are living in the now; this is something that the sane person knows, but the neurotic does not realise while enmeshed in a dreamlike pseudo-existence' (Naranjo, 1972, p. 77).

The difficulty with all needs-based theories is that of distinguishing needs from compulsions. For Gestalt theorists, if your recognition of your own feelings is faulty (if you mistake a feeling of self-doubt as the need for a doughnut or three) the cycle will not complete itself: you won't be able to 'bask' because the need will not feel met. Unfinished business (a concept all humanistic psychology uses in one form or another) is understood as requiring energy to push it down. There is a clear parallel here with the psychoanalytic concept of repression.

The main factor interfering with healthy development is the 'shoulds' emanating from society:

> In the early stages of development, the sense of identity is derived from the responses one gets from important and significant persons who, in some ways, serve as a mirror in which one sees oneself and from which one constructs an identity. This identity may be ill-formed or far removed from what one might really be when the authentic self is allowed to emerge and given the nourishment it needs. (Korb, Gorrell and Van De Riet, 1989, p. 46)

For Perls and other Gestaltists the healthy movement is from dependence to independence. The Gestalt prayer: 'You are you and I am I, and if by chance we find each other it's beautiful, if not it can't be helped' can be read as an injunction to take back projections and be clear about our boundaries. It can also be read as a denial of our real interdependence and a credo of egocentric individualism (Clarkson, 1989, p. 25). Gestalt has its own 'shoulds': you *should* live in the present, stop unnecessary thinking, take full responsibility for your feelings and actions and accept no shoulds (Naranjo, 1972, p. 57).

Both Rogers and Perls are open to the criticism levelled at all humanistic psychology: that it thinks of the inner or real self as pre-formed in accordance with human nature and of society as the cultural medium which either nourishes or stultifies this pre-given self, but does not construct it. The most socially critical – and socially optimistic – of our theories of human nature are arguably the most sociologically naïve. Maslow attempts to pre-empt this criticism by describing human nature as raw material 'rather than finished product, to be reacted to by the person, by his significant others, by his environment, etc. ... This raw material very quickly starts growing into a self as it meets the world outside and begins to have transactions with it' (Maslow, 1968, p. 190). This intrinsic nature of ours consists of potentialities rather than actualities. It is 'very easily drowned out by learning, by cultural expectations, by fear, by disapproval, etc.' (ibid., p. 191).

Maslow's theory of needs is widely invoked. It involves a hierarchy, in which higher needs are activated and begin to make their demands once basic needs are met. Basic needs can be recognized by gross effects of deficiency, such as illness. They are not all physiological: there are basic psychological needs for 'safety, belongingness, love, respect and self-esteem' (1968, p. 25). While these basic needs are unmet, we tend to regard people in terms of their use to us. When they are met, our motivational system switches into a higher gear and we start seeking 'self-actualisation' – moving towards fulfilling the possibilities intrinsic in our nature. In this model, the gratification of higher needs does not lead to 'basking' and diminution of appetite, except temporarily. The development of creativeness and understanding is itself rewarding. So good music may, by increasing our critical capacities, make us want more, even better music (Maslow, 1968, p. 30).

The notion of metal health Maslow develops on the basis of his memory of needs can justifiably stand in for humanistic psychology in general. Despite differences in detail, it represents the general thrust of the approach and the challenge it offers to psychoanalysis.

What is psychological health?

This challenge partly consists in the injunction to focus on positive health and its possibilities and to study examples of health.

> If we want to answer the question how tall can the human species grow, then obviously it is well to pick out the ones who are already tallest and study them ... If we want to know the possibilities for ... value growth or moral development in human beings, then I maintain that we can learn most by studying our most moral, ethical ... people. (Maslow, 1973, p. 7)

In other words good and healthy people are not exceptions in terms of their potential, but only in terms of the particular circumstances and choices which enabled them to realize it. They are not less, but more human than the rest of us – a position no psychoanalyst would take. Maslow argues that self-actualizers operate at a level, the B-level (B for being, contrasted with D for deficiency), where love is akin to thinking. We delight in the person, we see clearly what they are like, we may even be amused by or compassionate about their shortcomings, but we do not love for what we can get or what we can give. '[T]o the extent that perception is desire-less and fear-less, to that extent is it more veridical ... thus the goal of objective and true description of any reality is fostered by psychological health' (Maslow, 1968, p. 203).

Neurosis is not only a deficiency disease, but also a cognitive one. Healthy people are more in touch with reality, including moral reality; they have more access to their unconscious mind than less healthy people – they are able fearlessly to regress at will and they are in touch with their creativity. Finally, healthy B-motivated people often have 'peak experiences' of delight and awe. Rogers and other humanistic psychologists have also described healthy 'fully-functioning' people in detail, a project psychoanalysis never undertook. Rogers emphasizes that people who have moved towards 'the good life' as a result of psychotherapy or counselling would be insulted to be described as 'adjusted' (Rogers, 1990, p. 411). What they do have in common is flexibility, the lack of inner restrictions on choice; awareness of feelings, including unpleasant and painful ones; and the increasing tendency to live in the moment. Striving to meet our basic needs – our species requirements – brings out what all humans have in common. Striving towards self-actualization we become motivated by our own, individual nature; more idiosyncratic:

> the deficiency motivated man must be more afraid of the environment, since there is always the possibility that it may fail or disappoint him . . . In contrast, the self-actualising individual, by definition gratified in his basic needs, is far less dependent . . . self-directed. Far from needing other people, growth-motivated people may actually be hampered by them . . . The determinants which govern them are now primarily . . . the laws of their own inner nature. (Rogers, 1990, p. 35)

Compare Perls' notion of maturation as reduced dependence on 'shoulds' (Korb, Gorrell and Van De Riet, 1989, p. 46).

These are themes which recur again and again in humanistic descriptions of healthy people and the goals of therapy (e.g. Bonner, 1967, p. 61). They seem suspiciously culture-bound. Healthy people are said to reject convention, yet they implicitly obey a Western convention in being independent, self-reliant and autonomous. It sounds rather as if the self-actualizing individual becomes increasingly unaware of their dependence on their social and natural environment – less worried about the wherewithal and more about the details of the exhilarating sport of windsurfing. Yet Maslow denies that 'B-motivated' people are selfish. Another obvious problem is that the 'self-actualiser' is supposed to have transcended 'deficiency needs'. Artists must surely be self-actualizers, yet they have famously often been, like Van Gogh or Rodin, hungry, neurotic, yearning for love, yet continuing to obey their 'creative impulses'. 'Peak experiences' mark another anomaly. Maslow believed that these happened to self-actualizing people. Rowan describes how upset Maslow was at the LSD culture which offered ecstasy as an answer to boredom or depression (Rowan, 1988, p. 248). Maslow half meets these points when he talks of:

> a kind of pseudo growth . . . when the person tries (by repression, denial, reaction formation, etc.) to convince himself that an ungratified basic need has really been gratified or doesn't exist. He then permits himself to grow on to higher-need-levels, which of course . . . rest on a very shaky foundation such that the ungratified need remains as an unconscious force leading to various sorts of neurotic repetition. (Maslow, 1968, p. 58)

For Maslow's schema to be plausible this would have to be the commonest outcome. It highlights the inadequacy of the twin ideas of rigid levels and a relatively undifferentiated self. Most worrying, though, because of its political implications, is the implication that those who are materially deprived are necessarily psychologically unhealthy, stuck at the level of searching for gratification of their deficiency needs. Most of Maslow's 'highly evolved' B-cognizers seem to be professionals, businessmen, artists or homemakers and mothers married to men in these groups, in middle-class North America. We are not told whether they found their work (to which they are ideally suited) before or after becoming a self-actualizer (Maslow, 1973, p. 328). As we shall see in the next chapter, such deficit models of the complex link between health and social injustice dog needs-based theories of psychological health and ill-health.

Humanistic psychology clearly distinguishes 'positive health' from conformity. Despite its difficulties, it offers a clear model of human development and pathology, oriented towards human possibilities rather than their limits. Politically, it is an odd mixture. It is conservative, in that it maintains that however appalling the social situation, the road to self-actualization is possible. It is radical, in that it openly rejects conventional ideas (or at least some of them) about relationships and everyday behaviour. It is also radical in that it thinks the worst aspects of human behaviour and mental suffering result from bad early experience, with the implication that social reform could radically improve mental health. Would the relatively healthy then concern themselves with campaigning for such reforms? Some believe they would and do (e.g. Hampden-Turner, 1970; and Maslow himself came round to this position: 1976, p. xii). Others put the emphasis elsewhere. For the voluntarist basis of humanistic psychology can result in individualism or quietism, recourse to the inner changes of meditation, peak experiences and drug experiments that leave social structure just as it was. An example from the Gestalt writer Naranjo verges on the grotesque: 'at depth, we are where we want to be ... even when it amounts to apparent tragedy. If we can discover our freedom within our slavery, we can also discover our essential joy under the cover of victimisation' (1972, p. 78).

Certainly humanistic psychology criticizes and explains denial and conformity. But to see whether and how it can support active environmental politics, we need to look at its approach to my second question: What is the relationship between psychic structures and social structures?

Psychic structures, social structures

Humanistic psychology counterpoises individual and society, as did Freud. But where Freud saw society as taming the individual through the process of construction of the self and neurosis as an unfortunate side-effect of that necessity, Maslow *et al.* see social construction of the self as generally pathological. Social structures remain untheorized, indicated only by the term 'culture', which focuses on the realms of values rather than political and economic structures. Culture is seen as merely restricting (though in the Good Society it would enable). True, Maslow recognizes that culture is 'a *sine qua non* for the actualisation of humanness itself, e.g. language, abstract thought, ability to love; but these exist as potentialities in human germ plasm prior to culture' (Maslow, 1968, p. 211). He sees culture as a gardener who either fosters or inhibits growth. A better analogy would be the soil itself, for human beings cannot exist, let along grow, outside of culture, which must therefore be enabling even as it restricts.

Maslow refers to Mozart's creative potential, which his social environment fostered. But had Mozart been adopted at birth by Australian aboriginal people, he might or might not have become a master of the didgeridoo, but he would not have written 'Don Giovanni'. 'Don Giovanni' was not imprinted in his DNA, waiting for the cultural gardener to water it to fruition. There is more than a suggestion here of the individual's potentials as pre-formed fixtures. The effects of viewing the self as unitary and pre-formed are described by Frosch in a critique of object-relations theory for its 'humanistic' standpoint: 'the whole-ego argument also leads to an assertion of a fundamental separation of individual from society; the individual's psychic potential is pre-given, and it is the role of society simply to support that as it unfolds' (Frosch, 1987, p. 109). Maslow's implicit individual-society split is revealed in the statement that 'psychology is not reducible to sociology, because its unique jurisdiction [is] . . . that portion of the psyche which is not a reflection of the outer world or a moulding to it' (Maslow, 1968, p. 185). From a critical realist point of view there is a confusion of levels here. Even though causally generative structures at the level of mind *are* irreducible to structures at other levels, the 'outer world' co-determines the *effects* of the psychological structures. The psyche itself (like the phenotype) is always multiply determined and we infer the irreducible causally generative structures from the phenomenal confusion of effects.

The humanistic individual/society split leaves society – or culture – free-floating, its iniquities inexplicable since they are clearly nothing to do with human nature. Our genetic inheritance, as humans and as individuals, becomes a fixed term. Our human nature explains our similarity, our individual nature explains our differences. Culture is only causally effective in pathology. In such dichotomies as instinctual/learned, individual/society, explanation often proceeds by illegitimately treating one term as fixed. It is then thought of as the *essence* of the object of study and variation is due to the other mobile term. In humanistic psychology we have a similar explanatory mechanism working through three terms. We can use the analogy of a fruit-machine. On the left is human nature – say a lemon. This never goes round. In the middle is individual nature – lemon 1, lemon 2 and so on, all the possible forms of lemonness to infinity. However, in this machine the second lemon has a tendency to *look like* the third fruit, the social – say, a cherry. The social is constantly nudged by the mysterious process of history (*very* mysterious in this model) and spins round, sometimes showing a cherry, sometimes an orange, until that longed-for moment when it coincides with human nature, we have a row of lemons and we hit the jackpot for mental health. What we need is some idea of how to bring about this happy synergy.

Maslow concludes that neurosis is a deficiency disease, but fails to look at the systematic discrimination which ensures that some groups' basic needs are never met and that others benefit from this deprivation. At most Maslow acknowledges that

distributive inequality and other forms of injustice are widespread. It is this striking gap that allows him to reduce social structures, and the divisions and inequalities they involve, to the undifferentiated category of culture. In his study of people
who really are 'self-actualising', he notes that they are a tiny proportion of the population, but does not ask from which groups they come and what made it possible
for them to be as they are. As a result of these omissions, we are left with the
idea that, whatever our circumstances and history, if we aspire to the same atti-
tudes and approach as the B-cognizers, we can be like them by an act of will. On
the one hand, bad culture produces conformity, with its destructive effects on the
environments and our own mental wellbeing. On the other hand, the solution is in
our own hands.

Is there any virtue in this humanistic voluntarism, of which Gestalt represents
one of the more extreme versions? For Gestalt simply refuses to address the question of aetiology. Perls believes that causal explanations mix up 'memories and
history' (Perls, 1972, p. 18) and that this constitutes 'the great danger of the Freudian approach. "This happens because it has happened before." As if one railroad
station could be explained because there was another one before it' (op. cit., p. 33).
Similarly: 'Delving into the past serves the purpose of finding "causes" – and thus
excuses – for the present situation' (Perls, Hefferline and Goodman, 1951, p. 38).
Perls talks of our complete responsibility, which he spells response-ability, and our
infantile refusal to accept it. He often sounds rather like Szasz, who argues that
there should be no psychiatric pleas in law courts and no compulsory confinement
in mental hospitals (Szasz, 1974). But choice must be at the level of consciousness, or awareness in Gestalt terminology. Of what we are not aware, can we be
responsible? Perls would definitely say yes, for we are choosing to be unaware.
Whatever our reasons, it is a choice. Unconscious reasons, past real events, may
furnish explanations, but can neither rob us of choice nor provide justifications.

The question Perls and other humanists force us to confront is: Am I obliged
by my compulsion to eat these five Penguin biscuits, or do I choose? On a common
philosophical view, choice is integral to action. If I choose, if I scan my reasons,
evaluate them and act on the basis of that evaluation it is an action; if not, it is mere
behaviour (Milligan, 1980, p. 91). Psychoanalysts would extend the meaning of
action to cover behaviour motivated by unconscious as well as conscious wishes,
so that sometimes the former prevails and consciously controlled choice is unavail-
able to us. Humanistic psychologists would have it that we choose, we decide and
we can redecide.

They are right to classify compulsive actions as intentional, but they tend to
simplify the process of choice. The midwife tells the woman in transition not to
push yet, lest she damage the cervix. The woman now has a powerful reason for
waiting, as well as a powerful urge to push. The flasher has an overwhelming urge
to expose himself. Need he be overwhelmed? If there are no counter-reasons in
his awareness, that reason (the urge) will become causally effective – and he'll do
it. But if he knows the man up the road is a policeman in plain clothes, he may not.
If such another reason can affect what he does at a given moment, we are certainly talking about intentional action. The paradox disappears when we realize that

unconscious forces represent extremely strong reasons for acting, even though they offer at most a weak justification for it. In that sense we can do no otherwise, until insight gives us some counter-reasons to put in the balance, or actually weakens the pull. *Formally* we have a choice, as the action comes under the rubric of intentional. But actually we will not choose otherwise, cannot be expected to – any more than anyone can be expected to refrain from going to the toilet if their bladder is uncomfortably full. To the extent that Gestalt therapy sometimes seems to deny this, it is being naïve.

The common desire to be accepted within our social environment takes both conscious and unconscious forms and results in our framing our goals within its terms. Day by day, minute by minute, we are offered by the 'common sense' of our social environment, good reasons for continuing to act in ways that damage its natural foundations. Although these are unintentional actions, so that formally we always have a choice, we cannot be expected to do otherwise, unless we have some potent counter-reasons to put in the balance. These would need to challenge commonsense and to offer alternative ways of thinking and living on a wide scale. While individual choice has a significant role here, the strategic thinking which could provide these counter-reasons needs to come first in most cases. Certainly awareness of possible choices must play a role both in facilitating strategic thinking and in deciding to take non-obvious paths. Just as to focus on what you are aware of increases the scope of your awareness, focusing on the choice you exercise probably increases your ability to contemplate and evaluate the whole range of reasons which are likely to affect your action and to reduce your non-accidental 'forgetting' of certain options. Humanistic psychology may well have a contribution to make here.

However, this emphasis on strategy is my import rather than native to humanistic psychology. Rowan, for instance, in his recent overview of the field, endorses ecofeminist injunctions to awareness:

> The planet, Gaia, and the universe are now teaching us humans directly, nudging us along in the direction we must change, reconnecting us with the most fundamental living force, the urge to become all we can be, to evolve and to love it. We have this optimal program encoded in the proteins of our DNA. We *know* how to be healthy, how to cooperate as well as compete. These are older, deeper programs than our cultural programming. We are learning to tune back into them and to Nature, our surest teacher. (Henderson, 1982, quoted in Rowan, 1988, p. 230)

Again our own nature seems to provide the answer, if only we need it. Back to that fruit-machine – but this time it seems that if through awareness we succeed in getting a lemon in the middle, the social can be pulled (or nudged) into citric obedience.

After this, Rogers' approach, naïve as it is, seems almost politically astute. For several decades he maintained that 'person-centred' counselling was politically neutral. In his old age he came to see it as entailing certain political beliefs and values and ruling out others – and also as having potential for conflict resolution in the service of peace. He travelled to Northern Ireland, South Africa and other conflict-torn countries using his simple therapeutic model. In this the therapist, who needs to have a genuine attitude of 'unconditional positive regard' towards the client, listens uncritically to what the client says, replying by summing up the meaning and feelings the client has communicated. This reflective summing up indicates the therapist's non-judgemental acceptance of whatever has been said and allows the client to become more aware of their own feelings and to reveal further layers. In groups, the expression of feelings and the respectful listening to them should lead to the development of empathy and the search for common interests and creative solutions. Over time this approach would bring about social change by overthrowing prejudice, so that in increasing numbers the individual citizen:

> is not manipulated by powerful leadership . . . is enabled to become more
> of self . . . and it is out of that more complete and powerful humanness
> that person touches person, communication becomes real, tensions are
> reduced . . . this is the end result of a person centred politics in intergroup
> frictions. (Rogers, 1990, p. 445)

If there were two thousand such groups in Belfast, he suggests, real change could occur.

However valuable Rogers' belated attention to the dangers of denial in relation to nuclear war (1990, p. 446) and his work on intergroup conflict, with regard to social structures he remained naïve. Like most US humanistic psychologists, he could envisage changes in culture, values and traditions, but had no real concept of social structures, of interest groups and the institutions which represent them. For this reason his idea of how society causes human distress is a narrow one. Society is castigated for its failure to provide the relationships and values we need, but there is no analysis of the systematic disadvantaging of particular groups. Since the early 1970s the human potential movement has taken on the implications of gender inequalities and to some extent issues of ethnicity. But in doing so it has focused on feelings, values and individual actions rather than the institutional structures of sexism and racism. Unsurprisingly, it failed to extend itself to class, that bugbear of American life. Rowan, a modern British writer, represents the weaknesses of its approach:

> We have already seen that humanistic psychology can handle very well
> the conflicts between management and unions, black and white races,
> gender opponents, teachers and students . . . Why should it not be able
> to handle class conflicts too, so long as these are expressed in terms of
> genuine demands for real needs? In fact, this outlook should make class
> conflict more frequent and more productive. (Rowan, 1988, p. 238)

There is no distinction here between (1) psychotherapeutic work on the internalized effects of structural inequalities; (2) mediation and negotiation; and (3) moves to change the structure itself. Worse, there seems a suggestion that with the right psychotherapeutic tools, structural changes are redundant.

For humanistic psychology, the existence of 'violent and greedy behaviour' does not preclude a society which meets the basic and higher needs for all, if institutional arrangements can be devised in which 'the individual by the same act and at the same time serves his own advantage and that of the group' (Maslow, 1973, p. 210). Such 'synergy' makes self-actualization easier and allows the eventual transcendence of the very dichotomy selfish/unselfish through identification with other community members. This useful notion has been taken up within green movements, as we shall see. However, the poverty of humanistic conceptions of the relationship between psychological and social structures prevents it offering clues as to how to interrupt the social reproduction of environmentally destructive practices. It provides the notion of synergy, but unless we have some grasp of the workings of current anti-synergic forces and our collusion with them, no strategic conclusions can be drawn.

Chapter 8

Four radical approaches

Introduction: Lines of demarcation

The key feature of psychoanalytic thought, we have seen, is its emphasis on the aetiological role of unconscious processes. On the one hand the unconscious acts as a resource of energy and creativity, constitutive of society. On the other, it is a constant internal saboteur that undermines its most valuable creation – the rational thinking moral subject – and diverts human action into the repetitive compulsions emanating from destructive aspects of the drives. For Lacan, the 'rational thinking moral subject' is illusory from the beginning.

All would agree that the yearning for harmony within the self and between self and other, self and society, rests on an dangerous dream; for the pursuit of lost unity must involve the denial of reality and the use of projection:

> various people or concepts can be used as screens for such projections (the Jews, the bourgeoisie, patriarchal or industrial society, for example) and, because they are felt to be an obstacle to the realisation of the illusion, have to be ruthlessly annihilated. So murder is committed in the name of the ideal. (Chasseguet-Smirgel and Grunberger, 1986, p. 16)

At its starkest this view becomes fiercely reductionist. Chasseguet-Smirgel and Grunberger, in their lengthy diatribe against Reich, reject *any* causal role for social structure: 'human beings can only act, and create, on the basis of their internal, psychosexual model. We project this model out on to the world when creating political systems, institutions and economic structures, thus making them in our own image' (op. cit., p. 213). For them, analysis at the level of politics affords it a spurious autonomy, defensively denying 'the connections between the human psyche and its creations' which:

> seem to escape from their creators, becoming independent creatures . . . which invade from the outer world and mould the human psyche . . . At the heart of all ideologies lies the romantic and fashionable idea of

> 'changing the world'. Psychoanalytic understanding tends to act against this idea. (ibid.)

Resistance to this truth is inevitable, since it painfully 'confronts man with his own drives, deprives him of the outlet of projection, and makes him give up certain hopes' (1986, p. 214).

As for oppressive social relations, certainly our personal and collective struggles may have been made harder and more poignant by external events (as Shengold put it, we all have our holocausts (Malcolm, 1984, p. 84)). In this view, the conditions under which we live and work, the various groups we belong to – male, female, class, national and ethnic – and the experience which our group membership made us likely to have, do no more than provide the symbolic discourse within which we live out our own version of the Oedipal drama or the struggles of the paranoid-schizoid position. History has become an epiphenomenal and meaningless tapestry, a thousand ways of telling a single story. That our latest ways of acting out our timeless internal drama may destroy us is a mere contingency.

But unlike these authors, most psychoanalytic thinkers believe social structures do have relative autonomy and co-determine the formation of the self, within the broad template of intra-psychic processes. It is Society rather than societies that makes us ill. This illness cannot be reformed away because it is just an extreme form of normal development. Nevertheless it can be minimized, it can be contained, its symptoms can be diverted to relatively harmless forms. Political change is one of the keys to this. However, if politics is to avoid committing murder in the name of an ideal, it must be carried out from a 'healthy' position. This involves recognizing and taking responsibility for one's own destructive feelings without acting them out, while drawing on the positive, linking emotions of Eros (in the Freudian version) or love and gratitude (in the Kleinian).

Responsibility is a key word. For psychoanalysis, whatever the world did to us, we met it from the reservoir of our own desires. Were we sexually abused as a child? That was a serious difficulty. But the path to insight lies not in focusing on how power relations between women and men, sexism and heterosexism, make such episodes inevitable and simultaneously veil their normality, but in acknowledging how our own desire conditioned our response. Were we hungry? That too was something that should never have happened. But the key thing is not to focus angrily on the oppressive social relations which brought about our deprivation, but to take responsibility for what we made of the accidents of our upbringing and how we made ourselves in response. This can only be understood in terms of our own oral drives (in the Freudian version) or our own introjective urges, innate greed and envy (in the Kleinian one). Our present environmental malaise is not a direct result of ancient oppression and hurt, but the result of the ancient and modern feelings stemming from our instinctual inheritance – greed and aggression.

The therapeutic process in psychoanalysis involves retracing the steps of the construction of the self, with its current malaise and limitations. The stories told in the psychoanalytic consulting-room spell out what the person, in all their multiplicity, wanted, dreamed of and hoped to bring about, including the wishes they made sure they were unaware of. The aim is to restore the complexity to the person and thus to expand agency by making available – and bearable – the full richness of their inner dimensions. In this process society, which sets the manifest agenda, is taken as given. Not as perfect, but as given. Concentration on its imperfections may appear as a cop-out in relation to the often painful process of exploring the overdetermined levels of meaning that underlie our everyday activity.

Such a clear vision of inner reality necessitates a certain freedom from social convention, to which our passionate everyday desire is anathema. But while psychoanalysis may foster inner non-conformity, it also sets value on the ability and even the tendency to conform outwardly as an index of mental health. This is hardly stated, but is a palpable part of psychoanalytic culture. Jones knew Ferenczi loved Freud and (in theory at least) did not disapprove, but he did disapprove of Ferenczi enthusiastically embracing Freud after years of separation and division by war (Jones, 1953, p. 17). For Jones, this episode was one more nail in the coffin of Ferenczi's instability.

Similarly, in psychoanalytic circles, to be aware of one's homosexual feelings and to remain unphased by them is healthy; to act on them is not. There is some way in which heterosexuality is seen as *prima facie* evidence of mental health, as is the capacity to succeed in work, to hold down a good job. To be aware of the threat to the environment, to be concerned, to join pressure groups, is healthy; to decide there is no point at this moment in history, in doing anything other than try to save the planet is not. To have powerful feelings and to know one has them is healthy, but to cry in public or otherwise offend against the cultural ethos of self-control is not. To disapprove of discrimination against women or black people is healthy, but to become very angry about it is not. In other words, psychoanalysis does recognize that society needs changing, that while mental health is achievable (in its terms) as things are, it would be more readily so and would be so for more people if things were otherwise. But despite the need for social change, in general, psychoanalysis tends to be suspicious of the inability or refusal to conform. Here Lacan scores, for he places no premium on conformity. But since his theory provides no grounds for political commitment, it cannot endorse the passion of Earth First!

The disagreements between psychoanalysis and humanistic psychology are relatively well-known. Basic lines of demarcation are around whether the unconscious is timeless and universal or whether it is itself a product of specific social environments, which its contents reflect. As we have seen, the latter position is held not only by humanistic thinkers but, to varying degrees and in various respects, by such psychoanalytic theorists as Horney, Erikson and Winnicott. Similarly the line-up is not entirely straightforward around that other and related line of demarcation which divides those who believe a Good Society is possible from those who would settle for a better one.

No humanistic thinker holds a view analogous to that of Chasseguet-Smirgel and Grunberger. The closest would be the view of some of the older forms of Transactional Analysis, that Culture itself (rather than cultures) produces our malaise, our feelings of 'not-OK', and that we could not live without defensive scripts. But the middle ground, where most psychoanalysts and psychodynamic therapists are situated, allows for considerable and sometimes surprising convergence between psychoanalysis and humanistic psychology. Although Perls, for instance, berates psychoanalysis for its explanatory stress on causality, his own requirement of 'response-ability' in the present is not so far from psychoanalytic ideas of mental health. And while humanistic psychologies tend to emphasize the value of the independence of social convention, they have their own alternative culture and set of conventions of which they are less aware. Superficially the culture of the growth movement is very different from that of psychoanalysis, but there are similarities: most obviously a tendency to individualism, to see individual change as the primary route to social change.

This 'middle ground' is, essentially, the ground of therapy. Those who inhabit it may believe that politics serves a purpose, even a necessary purpose, but will see political process as largely separate from therapy, though it could usefully learn from it. Meanwhile, however pathogenic our societies, we can achieve a degree of mental health within them, a degree of competence and capacity to face reality. That is the task of therapy. The task of politics is to change social structures so as to bring them more in line with the best aspects of human nature. These tasks are related, but not inextricably intertwined. For some in the middle ground, education in matters psychological is the main focus of their hopes for political change, either because of their optimism about therapy and/or the early family and school environment, or because of their pessimism about political process. For these reformers, if parents, teachers and policy-makers were more in touch with their own feelings and had more understanding of the feelings of those in their charge, there would be no need for so many daily predictable disasters. Others, like Hanna Segal and Joel Kovel, see the need for specifically political action as well. The middle ground shades into the radical, as instantiated by the recently established British organization 'Psychotherapists and Counsellors for Social Responsibility', which says in a leaflet advertising its public launch:

> Many psychotherapists and counsellors are aware of a gap that can exist between their work with individuals or small groups and their concerns for wider social, cultural, racial and political issues. There is a sense in which what we have learned together as a profession is unnecessarily and damagingly confined to the clinical context. (PCSR, November 1995)

Jungian Andrew Samuels conducted a survey of analysts and psychotherapists in 14 organizations in 7 countries. He wanted to see whether colleagues would endorse his own feeling that patients were increasingly bringing political material into sessions and how they dealt with such material. Of the 14 organizations, 8 were Jungian, 1 (British) humanistic, 3 psychoanalytic (2 British and 1 US) and 1 (Russian) mixed (Samuels, 1993, p. 211). I cannot do justice to his interesting discussion here, but it suggests (on the basis of a 32 per cent response rate) that the gulf between humanistic and psychoanalytic therapists may not be so wide. For instance, in answer to the question: 'How do you deal with political material?', 65 per cent of the British psychoanalysts mentioned the symbolic and intra-psychic dimension

of such material – but so did 53 per cent of the humanistic practictione
believed in taking the material *only* on this level: 'The only way is to un
what is behind the political dimension and interpret it. Only that' (British psychoanalyst, quoted in Samuels, 1993, p. 237).

However, far more respondents mentioned exploring the meaning of the
material (*why* it was a concern for the patient, why now) and overall 71 per cent
mentioned the 'reality' of the patient's political concerns. Unsurprisingly, British
humanistic psychotherapists, British Jungians and US psychoanalysts were far more
likely to do so than British psychoanalysts (87 per cent, 86 per cent, 83 per cent
and 40 per cent respectively). But even this 40 per cent is surprising as suggesting the middle-ground is highly populated, especially when supported by such
remarks as: 'Over some universal and immoderately threatening issues such as
Chernobyl and the Gulf War . . . I would feel that it would be a mark of health
if a patient raised it and feel it is worrying if a patient does not do so' (British
psychoanalyst, quoted in Samuels, 1993, p. 237).

The implications of this remark are very relevant to radical therapy, as we
shall see. To his further questions: 'Do you find yourself discussing political issues
with your patients/clients? If not, why not?' Samuels once more got a surprising
number of analysts and therapists saying that they did (33 per cent of British psychoanalysts, 55 per cent of British Humanistics) as well as some outrage at having
been asked, from those who considered such discussion completely inappropriate.
Samuels concludes that there is indeed a split within the profession of analysis
and psychotherapy, 'between those who apprehend the reality of the political and
those whose definition of their job concentrates more on what is theorised as part
of the inner world' (Samuels, 1993, p. 26). There is also a further split, which he
sees as both promising and dangerous, between:

> the *public* apolitical, hyperclinical face of the profession . . . and the *pri-*
> *vate* face of the profession – practitioners all too aware they have political
> histories themselves, struggling to find a balance between inner-looking
> and outer-looking attitudes to what their patients bring to them. (ibid.)

The middle-ground shades into the radical, for whom societies, rather than Society,
are to blame for psychological distress and ill-health. These thinkers are clear that
health-as-normal-functioning and conventional success in our present societies can
only be obtained at the expense of at least some aspects of positive health. They
believe the unconscious is partly socially formed and itself plays a political role.
For them, real psychological health must therefore involve social criticism, with
the corollary that the therapist cannot be politically neutral. They are more likely
to consider present-time anger an appropriate, even a useful response. Radicals
are dissatisfied with the conventional view that therapy is progressive because it
increases the net amount of health in a society. This conventional view suggests
that individual health is achievable in 'crazy' and destructive societies, which most
radicals consider problematic.

It also implies either that health is additive and social health can be reached once a certain critical mass of healthy individuals is reached; or that healthy individuals would routinely make political choices which bring social health nearer. For radicals, a psychologically distressed person (which includes us all, to various extents) needs to see through internalized untruths about themselves and about social relations, in order to get a better grasp of reality. But that better grasp will only be genuinely empowering if it involves practice. An accurate description of the social relations which have caused the person suffering in the course of their life entails their condemnation and an imperative to change them. This political act, on however small a scale, will be empowering – an 'acting out' of insight. Thus Marie Langer (1989) and her colleagues had at one point as part of their goals for group work at a hospital:

> to help our patients lose, or at least diminish, their sexual and social prejudices and to liberate themselves relatively speaking from the ideology of the dominant class ... to achieve unexpected revelations in the weakening of repression and unconscious guilt feelings [by helping them] discriminate between their responsibility for their personal history and that of their family and society. (Langer, 1989, p. 177)

Instead of health as normal functioning, we have health as radical critique; the internal freedom to work out and choose social revolution or other political steps which go far beyond therapeutic settings.

Power, knowledge and the aim of therapy

All radical social critics are likely to fall foul of the norms of mental health that play a crucial role in social reproduction. But not all political 'extremists', 'obsessionals', 'ecofreaks', 'weirdos' and 'fanatics' take up aspersions on their sanity as part of the struggle. Nor do they all feel that psychological damage has been inflicted on them and seek healing for it as part of their political practice. The labour movement and socialist left in particular have tended to perpetuate the conventional split between the personal and the political, seeking a reversal of values and change of power relations without recourse to any separate healing of injuries inflicted by class. In contrast the women's movement and sections of the anti-racist and anti-colonial movement have theorized the psychological effects of sexism, racism and colonialism, developing therapeutic practices informally linked to and supportive of these liberatory movements. To counter ruling ideas of health-as-normal-functioning, they have to relativize these and show them as non-obvious and non-natural. But to go further – as they must if their project is political change – they have to offer alternative notions of health and of the aim of therapy. In this section I draw on feminist therapy and transcultural therapy for examples, without being able to do justice in this small space to their diversity and depth.

The roots of feminist therapy lie in consciousness raising (CR) as developed in the Western women's liberation movement during the 1970s. CR challenged the received notions of social reality, which inevitably raised mental health issues. Such is the power of 'normal functioning' as a criterion of sanity that it is hard to challenge it in thought as well as in practice. In a slave society, it is hard to see slaves as fully human people who are mistreated even when they are 'treated well'. Similarly, the 'normality' of male domination makes it hard to see. Against this cultural background some defences against psychic pain are visible and look odd or 'crazy', while others look perfectly normal and well-adjusted. For example, paranoia is more visible than its obverse: the idea that people are treating you well when they are actually behaving in a hostile manner. Much of women's 'normal functioning' was later to be seen by feminist therapists as a defence against the anger and loss they would have to feel if they recognized the full size of sexism. It was this defence that came under attack through the practice of CR.

CR worked by making the personal public, recasting the 'inadequate' or 'guilty' woman as victim and survivor of oppression: 'the public revelation of the many and ancient sexual secrets of women (orgasm, rape, abortion) may have contributed far more toward the liberation of women than the attempt to heal individual wounds through a restorative therapeutic relationship' (Herman and Hirschman, 1984, p. 256). It named sexism as a non-natural set of oppressive practices, in which men were the perpetrators and women (often) the colluders. This challenge required somewhere else to stand and the proposed foundation was at first *experience* – women's experience, up to now considered insignificant or shameful. Feminist therapy initially inherited this emphasis on experience: the strength and the weakness of CR. Lipschitz, an early psychoanalytic critic of feminist therapy, wrote:

> For an analyst, experience cannot be truth because ... [it] is only part of the story always. However, feminist therapy and consciousness raising groups assume this in their use of the consensual validation of individual experience. Not only is the group seen as a microcosm of collective social experience, but the individual is in turn seen as merely reflecting cultural experience in general. (1978, p. 25)

In fact, CR groups were highly selective. Whereas psychoanalysis could ignore, as immaterial to its object, the extent to which the female patient's experience was structurally and culturally determined, CR only validated those individual experiences which could plausibly be seen as reflecting women's collective social position. This empiricism was a necessary stage in which women's hidden experiences were temporarily fetishized under pretence of respect for *all* female experience. It was an unsustainable position for a therapeutic practice, although remnants of its rhetoric persist in some feminist therapy alongside positively authoritarian prescriptions. Thus Ballou and Gabalac insist that 'women's experience as felt, lived and processed is the trusted base for knowledge' (1985, p. 58) and that 'feminist therapy does not impose any model of health but rather seeks to assist women in evolving and developing their own' (ibid., p. 66); but ten pages later they are describing at length just what a healthy woman is like.

Experience must always be important to radicals, since the experience of marginalized groups tends to be silenced or denied. Feminist and transcultural therapists have explored two particular reasons for valorizing the patient's/client's experience as brought to the therapy relationship. First, in this asymetrical power relationship the experience of the patient/client is submitted to the therapist to be scrutinized, explored and given meaning. Or so it can feel. And the interpretation the therapist may assign to the experience may seem to the patient/client to deny its validity, to attribute feelings of abuse or oppression to inner rather than outer reality, to pathologize. In Siegel's first therapy, she claimed:

> my present concerns and activities were discounted and made invisible. The guilt and dependency were reinforced. The message was: if I stopped resisting and acting out, the neurosis could be cured and I would no longer be so unnecessarily depressed. I got through this difficult period, gradually replacing midlife mourning with midlife planning

but no thanks to the therapist (Siegel, 1983, p. 96).

Second, while the experience of the patient/client is made problematic, that of the therapist is denied salience. In this relationship the therapist is, in Lacan's phrase, 'he-who-is-supposed-to-know'. Paradigmatically male, he stands nowhere and everywhere on the objective ground of science, discounting his own experience, which must not enter the session except to the extent that his own feelings offer information about the patient's. Arguably even the therapist's awareness of the counter-transference leaves the power relation intact, since the onus is still on him to disentangle his patient's projections from his own, producing knowledge. This is the model that radical therapists reject; and a certain empiricism can follow from that rejection. However, it need not. All that need be said is that the therapist, too, is speaking and judging from experience, from a social position and to demand that that experience and that position be rendered visible. We can then ask whether the theory that is being used offers an account of *both* sets of experience (that of patient/client as well as that of therapist) and can explain their discrepancies; where the account leads, politically speaking; and whether it is recognizable and convincing to the patient/client according to shared and agreed-on criteria. Experience is no substitute for theory, but unless theory can deal with experience it is useless.

Humanistic psychology has far less difficulty with such modifications than does psychoanalysis. It sees the asymetrical therapy relationship as a temporary expedient where (theroretically at least) the positions could be reversed on some later occasion. Initially humanistic therapies were far more attractive to feminists seeking healing, because humanistic feminist therapies could assure their clients 'that what was wrong was the constraints of the stereotyped role . . . not her response' (Smith and Siegel, 1985, p. 18). Psychoanalysis made a comeback, though, when the limits of voluntarism were reached. Committed feminists who found themselves hating and competing with their 'sisters', or internally attached to fantasies of submission or dependence, found the concept of the unconscious offered a possible way of understanding oppression stemming from within.

> The feminist analysis of women's rage or dependence that blames it all on external society, as in the slogan 'women are not mad, they are angry', overlooks the internal struggle ... and ignores unconscious sources of self-defeating behaviour ... however painful, the acknowledgement of how women oppress themselves and others is ultimately liberating. What is unconscious can be made conscious. (Flax, 1981, p. 61)

For that reason, eclectic approaches have become popular in feminist therapy, approaches which recognize the unconscious and use the transference, but which also draw on humanistic techniques and ideas of the professional-client relationship.

Within psychoanalysis, feminist therapists have taken up wider debates about the transference and restated them in terms of women's psychology. They have become strong critics of classical and of Kleinian notions of the transference, claiming that it can perpetuate sexism. For example, Lerner claims that male therapists with female patients often collude with their presentations of themselves as dependent and passive: 'the weaker sex must protect the stronger sex from recognising the strength of the weaker sex lest the stronger sex feel weakened' (Lerner, 1984, p. 129). Such collusion ensures that the woman's unconscious anger remains buried.

Another point at issue has been the requirement that the analyst should not gratify the patient's unconscious desires, which some analysts understand as a prohibition against smiling or saying 'Good morning. How are you?' Some feminist therapists (including feminist object-relations therapists) argue that the model of 'analyst as blank screen' results in a failure to acknowledge the present relationship, which can lead to a negative infantilizing transference not unlike women's position in the social strucure (Greenspan, 1983, p. 238). They believe the resulting frustration simply repeats women's daily experience of putting aside their unmet needs and propose instead that appropriate present-time needs should be met within the therapeutic relationship (Greenspan, 1983, p. 247; Eichenbaum and Orbach, 1987, p. 62). Others deeply disagree (Lipshitz, 1978, p. 26; Bar, 1987, p. 252).

Transcultural therapy makes a similar challenge to the objectivity and universality of the transference and the therapy relationship. Originating in the meeting of medical anthropology and cultural psychiatry (Littlewood, 1990), it has intellectual roots in the dispute between Freud and Malinowski as to whether the Oedipus complex is universal (Malinowski, 1960). The Transcultural Psychiatry Society was set up in Britain in 1976 with the aim of increasing sensitivity towards cultural difference (Mercer, 1986, p. 118). By 1990, in the face of the disproportionate numbers of Afro-Caribbean people diagnosed as schizophrenic and their higher rates of compulsory admission to mental hospitals, such sensitivity was increasingly seen as requiring a commitment to anti-racism rather than 'multiculturalism' (McGovern and Cope, 1987, p. 510; Littlewood and Lipsedge, 1981, p. 270). As in feminist therapy, a range of techniques may be used, sometimes side by side (d'Ardenne and Mahtani, 1989). Sue and Sue (1981) argue that the choice of technique is part of the process, since some are more acceptable to people with particular cultural backgrounds. D'Ardenne and Mahtani give an example of a Nigerian man who found his white counsellor's 'neutral' facial expression cold and superior seeming (1989, p. 99). Yet these techniques are all justified by theories with universal claims.

There are particular difficulties with psychoanalysis, for transcultural therapy as for feminist therapy. Where the therapist is white and the client black, whatever the technique, the client has to decide to trust the therapist despite continuing bad experiences at the hands of the therapist's group. For this to be possible the client tends to test the therapist in various ways and a degree of self-disclosure is important – which rules out some versions of psychoanalysis (Sue and Sue, 1981, p. 71). Further, theories of transference recognize projective processes on both sides, but do not necessarily allow the role of race in these to become visible. For transferential processes are not merely individual or limited to therapeutic sessions: 'Inevitably there occurs a social and communal transference related to other individuals and other groups of people and this plays an important role in the encounter even for experienced analysts. Such feelings lie in a very primitive part of ourselves' (Kareem, 1992, p. 22). Yet psychoanalytic candidates are given no guidance in their training on working through such feelings (nor, for that matter, are trainee therapists and counsellors). Lastly, psychoanalysis does not readily allow the therapist to communicate 'that society can be wrong and can be responsible' or to refuse 'to offer solace to an individual at the potential price of leaving the group behind', preconditions according to some of successful psychotherapy with black people (Thomas and Comer, 1973, p. 175).

Feminist therapy and transcultural therapy reject the idea of value-free therapy and require the therapist to acknowledge their own experience, theory, assumptions and aims. Experience is various and relative, but therapy must have direction, despite attempts from diverse positions to suggest the therapist could and should have an open mind about outcome (Laing, 1960, p. 25; Bion, 1984, p. 151). Even if we trust the patient's 'wisdom of the organism', we must have theorized it sufficiently to be able to distinguish it from unwisdom when it does emerge. 'Central to every form of psychotherapeutic treatment are beliefs about what people are like and what they might become' (Sturdivant, 1980, p. 7). Such beliefs inevitably have political implications. Concepts of mental health are themselves gendered (Broverman, 1981; Lerner, 1984, p. 272) and 'raced' (Littlewood and Lipsedge, 1981, p. 253).

Therapists have always taken political positions, always made judgements about social reality: feminist and transcultural therapy have just made this more visible. For instance, a therapist considering taking on an unhappy middle-aged white housewife as a patient has to make several judgements before deciding whether to recommend therapy. They have to judge whether what they are being told is true (in the superficial sense: is the woman really a housewife, as she reports, or is this a fantasy? etc.). They have to judge the extent to which the woman's responses are appropriate reactions to her situation and the extent to which they can only be explained in intra-psychic terms. This calls for an understanding of the position of women – and housewives in particular – as well as the particular context of this woman's life. It calls for a position on human needs, including female human needs, and whether this social context allows this woman's needs to be met. The decision as to whether this woman's reaction is an expression of neurotic conflict or whether 'it is our very definitions of femininity and the feminine role that are a pathogenic cause of female symptomatology, has important clinical implications' (Lerner, 1984, p. 272). It is likely to be both. Differences on this axis might lead to emphasis on one of the two obvious questions: 'Why is the woman unhappy in this situation?' versus '(Given that anyone would be unhappy in this situation) why is she not changing it?'

Most of these judgements would be made by the therapist extremely quickly and sometimes below the level of awareness, especially if the woman comes from a similar social background. If the woman is Jewish (and the therapist is Gentile), if she is lesbian or bisexual and the therapist is not, or if she comes from a minority nationality and the therapist does not, the possibility of this cultural background being relevant to her malaise springs into view. Either the therapist attempts to ignore this difference ('colour-blind' or 'nation-blind' or 'religion'-blind therapy), or they now wonder whether an unfamiliar symbolic vocabulary is being invoked, or whether the actual social situation of the woman as a member of this group is a factor. But where therapist and patient are both from the dominant group, the relevance of this is unlikely to be thought about. Radical therapists require therapists to see people as members of groups, yet to do *only* this is also oppressive.

Transcultural therapists emphasize that the point of putting people in social context is precisely to allow their individuality to become visible, so that the black person is seen as having 'normal and ordinary' individual characteristics (Thomas, 1992, p. 134). Both feminist therapists and transcultural therapists insist that when people are being oppressed in the present this needs acknowledging within the therapeutic relationship – it cannot and must not *only* be treated as a pointer to early material, though it may be that too. For radicals the link between psychic and social structures is so close (each is mediated through the other) that oppressive social relations necessarily enter into the construction of the self and have to be recognized and countered in therapy.

Politics could be evident in termination criteria too. The traditional psychoanalytic aim is to make some unconscious feelings conscious and to achieve integration. Feelings of anger which had previously been unconscious could be recognized and accepted and ways found of living harmlessly with them or even harnessing them creatively. But what looks like integration and what looks harmless depend very much on whether you accept health-as-normal-functioning or whether you see such adjustment as itself destructive and pathological. For feminist and other radical therapies, achieving the degree of health which is possible in our present societies involves refusing to accept oppression and injustice and directing appropriate anger against them. Just as Fanon saw anti-colonial violence as itself therapeutic (1968), feminists have seen action against women's oppression essential part of healing.

y was angry at her father for his arbitrary and cruel power. She was also angry at her boss for his arbitrary and cruel power. In psychodynamic theory, the two figures ... are related only symbolically (within Amy's unconscious) rather than in reality ... [which circumvents] the question of the legitimacy of Amy's anger – both at her boss and at her father

writes one feminist therapist. She goes on:

both father and boss are not merely male authority figures in Amy's unconscious, but also real men ... linked ... institutionally by the two symmetrical social arrangements of male domination in which they rule: the nuclear family and the capitalist workplace. (Greenspan, 1983, p. 175)

Greenspan here justifiably stresses what psychoanalysis chooses to ignore: the similarities in social position of boss and father in the external world. But it would be disastrous to ignore what psychoanalysis stresses; for unless Amy can disentangle boss and father, ancient and present anger, she will not be able to act effectively and appropriately. As with Klein's notion of reparation, we have to distinguish the possible healing effect of particular political actions from their effectiveness in the world.

To sum up, radicals point out that therapists (and the theories they use) always take political positions which affect the course and the aim of therapy and that it is insidious and conservative to deny this. To the invisible, hegemonic positions they counterpose their own, which sees health as involving being able to distinguish between what we did and what was done to us. For those who have been and still are being oppressed, health must involve feeling appropriate anger about past oppression and taking steps to prevent its continuing in the present. In our societies this can only mean that political action is integral to psychological health.

Oppression is bad for your health

Both feminist and transcultural therapy start off with the assumption that oppression is pathogenic. In Western countries women and certain ethnic groups are overrepresented in the mental health statistics (Pilgrim and Rogers, 1993). Why? Is it because gendered and 'raced' notions of health 'see' women and people of colour as 'abnormal'? Or have oppressive social relations really taken their toll? Let us take the simpler case of gender. 'This relative excess of women occurs across almost all the diagnostic categories of psychiatry, with the exception of alcoholism and personality disorder, but is most marked in relation to depression and the psychoneuroses' writes Allen, (1986, p. 85). One obvious possibility is that men and women are treated differently by the mental health system. Broverman *et al.* found that US clinicians' ideas of a healthy man and a healthy adult were very similar, but their ideas of a healthy *woman* included submissiveness, dependence, lack of adventurousness, lack of objectivity, easily hurt feelings and so on – all incompatible with their ideas of healthy adulthood (Broverman, 1981, p. 95).

Some feminists have redescribed these characteristics as intelligent survival skills – yet have to recognize that they exact a costly penalty (Carmen, Russo and Miller, 1984, p. 21). Others have noted that concepts of maturity usually include separateness and autonomy – qualities that in Western societies come easier to men, rather than the equally necessary social capacity for close relatedness. Yet women's most common difficulty (reaching autonomy) is pathologized more than men's difficulty in getting close (Burch, 1985, p. 107). It seems likely both that women's oppression really does harm them psychologically and that women's resistance and unhappiness are inappropriately medicalized and judged according to gendered standards of mental health.

How could women's oppression make women sick? It might be the case that women's social position would make *anyone* sick. Marriage and motherhood could come into this category. Especially as experienced by working class women, they appear to make women vulnerable to depression and other forms of mental illness (Rieker and Carmen, 1984, p. 25). On one interpretation these women are unhappy because they are in a humanly impossible situation: that is, they would be unhealthy if they *were* happy, with the corollary that the 'adjusted' are really in worse shape (Howell, 1981, p. 509). This view falls into sociological reductionism when it suggests that women's mental ill-health is the mechanical and unmediated result of present adverse social circumstances (Ballou and Gabalac, 1985, p. 23). It also fails to distinguish between unhappiness and depression, so that the only real pathology becomes a tendency to self-blame which can be overcome through feminist education and solidarity. Now, much depression among mothers of young children could be due to the social organization of childcare, without it following that the depressed are really the healthy. A better starting point could be the work of Brown and Harris, which sees depression as a likely response to the extra stress caused by difficult life circumstances and lack of support, when this combines with the effect of early loss (1978, p. 279). People for whom daily life is a never-ending struggle are constantly up against their own vulnerability.

This first argument – Allen calls it the 'weak form' (1986, p. 91) – bypasses the question of how women's oppression affects the construction of the gendered self. Most feminist therapy has gone further, agreeing with Chesler (criticized by Allen, 1986, p. 95) that women really are sicker than men, but it is the male-imposed feminine role which has made them so. Chesler combines this 'deficit model' with labelling theory, so that women are both sicker (because of their internalization of the feminine role) and labelled as so. Women are diagnosed as mentally ill when they are *too* feminine, according to Chesler (depressed, hysterical, over-emotional) and as 'mad' when they reject femininity (Chesler, 1972, p. 53).

Without taking on all of Chesler's rhetorical and often confused account, most feminist therapists agree that the internalization of oppressive messages is devastating to women's mental health. To believe that something happens to you *because* you are 'beautiful' or 'ugly', that it is reasonable for a jealous man to hit, for a sexually 'provoked' one to assault, for an employer to patronize, is to accept social confirmation of early feelings of unworthiness and is fundamentally disempowering. Women who believe they deserve no more are likely to accept situations producing inner disturbance or conflict and to underestimate their individual or collective power to change these aspects of their lives (Miller, 1984, p. 48). 'Oppression has not just existed but has become part of our view of ourselves, and . . . must be brought to awareness in order for change to occur in ourselves and the world' (Lerman, 1985, p. 7).

To sum up, most feminist therapy holds that (1) women are systematically discriminated against, restricted and invalidated, which harms them psychologically as well as materially and socially. (2) Women's subordination enters into the construction of the self, which is even more harmful; and (3) the medicalization of women's unhappiness and rebellion and the reimposition of an oppressive normality through the mental health system, are themselves pathogenic. According to this view, both in 'mental illness' and in health-as-normal-functioning, women fall short of their own potential for positive health.

The analogy with transcultural therapy is a strong one, though it was stronger 50 years ago when the biological concept of race paralleled that of sex as providing 'natural' pretexts for inequality. Human beings really are sexed, however tenuous the connection between sexual difference and the practices it is used to justify, so the category of 'sex' survives its deconstruction. In contrast, the category of 'race' has been effectively debunked and most of its meanings shifted to the ambiguous terms 'culture' and 'ethnic group'. Anti-racism now has to counter the pretence that discrimination is an appropriate response to cultural difference. Since cultural difference is conceptualized as voluntary, in a classic blame-the-victim move inequality can be blamed on the inadequacy of the Caribbean or African American family, on arranged marriages, etc.

This can pose problems for transcultural therapy because of its own reliance on the concept of culture. Nevertheless, the parallels are striking. As feminist therapy identifies sexism as pathogenic, transcultural psychology claims that racism *causes* mental illness, both directly and indirectly. Littlewood writes: 'To be black in Britain today is to be exposed to a variety of adverse stimuli which can add up to quite a serious hazard to mental health (1992, p. 3). On an argument similar to that of Brown and Harris (1978), to be treated as inferior, to be hated, to be discriminated against, are sources of stress which increase the vulnerability to emotional distress rooted in early life (Bavington 1992, p. 103; Thomas, 1992, p. 138). As feminist therapy sees women's internalization of their social invalidation as psychologically harmful, so transcultural psychology claims that racism establishes an internal white racist in every black person, continually generating feelings of badness and worthlessness. As feminist therapy argues that the mental health system is itself sexist, transcultural therapists claim that it is racist (Mercer, 1986, p. 115).

In feminist therapy there is some tension between the position that women are fine and healthy *on their own terms* and the position that they are psychologically damaged by sexism. On the first position, exemplified by much ecofeminism, sexism devalues women's canonical qualities. Women's capacity for close relationships,

their non-violence, their intuition, their openness to emotions, their
tion – it would be a better world if these became the dominant v
tices. On the second position, we need to heal the split in human natu.
by gender divisions. There is some analogy between this debate and the tension in
transcultural therapy between (1) the cultural relativist view: that health is relative
to culture and the transcultural therapist's job is to accept the therapeutic aims
of the client's culture, if not of the client. Thus Littlewood called in Pentecostal
Church elders to decide whether a member of their church was speaking in tongues
or was mentally ill (Littlewood and Lipsedge, 1989, p. 174). (2) The anti-racist
view, that the therapist has to understand and communicate the role of racism in
order to help the client heal.

These might be compatible, if it were accepted that in a racist society there
is a particular need to re-establish the value of minority cultures. But there is considerable philosophical tension here. (1) draws on the views of Erikson (1965) and
Horney (1937) that the self is constructed within a culture as a result of its material
practices, especially child-rearing, and the meaning it gives to these. The trouble is,
it tends to assume that cultures are discrete, readily identifiable, static and internally
homogenous. It also assumes they can only be judged on their own terms. Thus
Littlewood and Lipsedge, who vacillate between (1) and (2), describe a delusion as
a false belief not sanctioned by one's culture (1981, p. 207). Thus Sue and Sue, firm
cultural relativists, describe black people 'playing the dozens' (exchanging taunts
and abuse) in functionalist terms, as a way – and by implication a good way – of
learning to 'take' abuse without expressing anger (1981, p. 66).

Such indiscriminate respect for cultures must surely result in conservatism
and has to accept culturally legitimated racist and sexist beliefs and practices. It
certainly precludes developing a notion of *human* positive health which can be
used as a basis for social criticism – as in (2). In taking equality of treatment as
a value for all cultures, (2) makes claims to universal validity. For anti-racism,
therapy can play an important supportive role to political action, and vice versa.
Therapy can be empowering, even if for the time being it is separate from political and economic change. Littlewood and Lipsedge discuss an example of a black
woman who felt her blackness as bad and dirty. They set the therapeutic goal of
helping her accept her own ambivalence:

> It may be objected that her difficulties are inherent in a racist situation
> and that our intervention only helps her to adjust to this ... If we can
> show her, however, the social origins both of her difficulties and also of
> the way by which she has tried to solve them, we are offering her a power-
> ful way to adjust reality to conform to her needs rather than the reverse.
> (1981, p. 238)

But the trouble for both anti-racist transcultural therapy and feminist therapy is
that they tend to fall into a deficit model. If you argue that oppression produces
mental illness, it may seem as though oppressing is good for your health. Middle-
class white people in the US, Britain, Canada and Australia are relatively free from

the stresses of racism, poverty and harassment. Have they cornered the mental health as well?

> The problems of the Black community were largely imposed on it by the oppressive exploitation of the white community. The health of the white community – in political, economic, educational and psychological terms – is based on the systematic production of white-generated and defined pathology within the Black community

wrote one black US mental health worker in the 1970s (Wilcox, 1973, p. 466). Were the SS guards, well-adapted to their culture, in better health than the Jewish inmates they tortured? Are men in better health than women? In the light of male violence and addictions it seems implausible that taking the oppressor role is good for your health (Pleck, 1984, p. 87; Miller, 1978, p. 88). The deficit model is a trap into which those who have done some of the most detailed work on the rela-tionship between internal and external sometimes tend to fall. For instance, (citing Chasseguet-Smirgel) Maguire (1987) speaks of the 'sense of incompleteness' found in infants of both sexes because of their overwhelming dependence on an all-powerful mother. 'Unlike boys, girls cannot compensate for these narcissistic wounds and assert their autonomy from their mothers by demonstrating that they have something which is not only different, but more highly valued in our society' (Maguire, 1987, p. 146). In the same volume, Orbach and Eichenbaum discuss and ultimately reject the view that 'feminine emotional values' are positive, which 'would seem to elevate a consequence of oppression into a virtue' (1987, p. 54). In fact, they say, the price paid for women's connectedness is the loss of the sense of self. 'Let's turn briefly to what women in therapy present, for there can be no more dramatic exposure of this tragic underbelly ... it is startling to realise quite how low women's self-esteem is' (ibid.). I have no reason to doubt this testimony. But are men any better off?

Beyond the deficit model

We turn now to two radical psychologies which have no truck with the deficit model. We will see in the concluding section and in the next chapter how relevant this is to 'ecopsychology', where all humans (to varying extents) can be seen as both oppressors and oppressed.

Re-evaluation Counselling is the original co-counselling, invented by Harvey Jackins and colleagues in the 1950s, in which 'people of all ages and ... back-grounds can learn how to exchange effective help with each other in order to free themselves from the effects of past distress experience' (cover of the quarterly magazine *Present Time*). It rejects the name of 'therapy', since it has neither profes-sionals nor experts and it insists on open, turn-taking peer-counselling relationships in a healing process in which every cog wheel is visible. It is organized in informal 'communities' in more than 50 countries, with their own accredited teachers and leaders. Loosely humanistic, in some respects it rejects humanistic liberalism. It has clear guidelines discouraging smoking, alcohol and other drugs and socializing with other co-counsellors and it has a clear leadership structure. Of all the theories I have looked at, Re-evaluation Counselling (henceforth RC) has absolutely no quasi-academic literature attaching to it. Harvey Jackins, a working-class trade-union militant of the 1930s, was determined that RC should not get confused with the plethora of growth-movement therapies or intellectualized out of the reach of ordinary people. It trains no professionals and spreads mainly by word of mouth, so it is rarely mentioned in print outside its own publications (Rowan, 1988, is one of several exceptions).

RC insists on its (humanistic) view that human beings are basically good – that is, pro-social: cooperative, loving, intelligent, flexible and enthusiastic. 'We do not have *bad* people; we have good people acting bad when they are short-circuited by the emotional scar tissue which has been loaded on them by the environment' (Jackins, 1965, p. 68). RC is in some ways the obverse of psychoanalysis. Psycho-analytic workers in private life are often uncomfortably suspicious of apparent love and harmony. They tend to pounce on evidence of negative feelings, the sinister side of human beings, as if this were *more real* than the loving side. Without denying the appalling ways in which human beings frequently behave, RCers simply award ontological priority the other way round. 'We do not have human beings with *inherent* conflicts which they must learn to live with; we have con-sistent human beings warped into apparent self-conflict by *acquired* distress patterns which act contrary to their inherent rational nature' (ibid.). These 'distress patterns' result from environmental failure.

For RC, basic human needs are universal, though they may be variously met. They include the chance to love and be loved, to form close, committed relation-ships, to receive and give respectful, affectionate touching and holding, to have physical needs met in a way that the person controls. The social environment, whatever it is, must allow the person to be creative and to be valued for it and it must provide a system of meanings which allows them to make sense of the world. Above all, it must provide attention from loving, aware people who retain the sense of their separateness as well as their connection. As in all needs-based theories, basic needs are recognizable by the deleterious effects of their neglect (cf. Doyal and Gough, 1991, p. 42).

All these needs are far more crucial for the developing child, who cannot know as adults can that 'She didn't really mean it' or 'That need will be met next Thursday'. Environmental failure leaves the child with the additional difficulty of reconciling its loving feelings about the caring adult, and its fear of loss, with its anger and grief (cf. Miller, 1983). According to RC, unless the child is allowed to heal through emotional discharge, rigid distress patterns will be set up by hurtful experiences. Hurting interferes with thinking, although the attempt to think does not stop. The details of the hurt become mis-stored as a rigid block, so that any one of them can, in future, evoke the whole experience and provoke the re-enactment of what happened (or was felt to happen), together with the feelings and frantic attempts at thinking that were going on. 'In the grip of the re-stimulated distress recording, the person talks foolishly, acts inaccurately and unsuccessfully, and feels terrible feelings that have no logical connection with what is actually going on' (Jackins, 1965, p. 48).

According to RC the patterns laid down in the past are 're-stimulated' most of the time and most adult emotion is a replaying of undischarged ancient feelings. Our habitual patterned responses are so 'chronic' that they are misunderstood as our 'personalities'. Even present-time hurtful events, like being robbed or raped, get most of their power to hurt from the earlier feelings. Adults have the power to get their needs met, or can at least attempt to change the social environment so that they can be met. Yet most of the time we behave powerlessly or addictively and these debilitating responses are echoes of childhood pain, a patterned mimicking of the dependency of infancy. We retain, if we are lucky, areas of flexible thinking and resource. Some cultures are more likely to allow resource in one area, some in another. But it is our chronic patterned thinking and feeling which makes us the tools and the instigators of social irrationality, including ecological destruction.

In some respects RC resembles other needs-based theories, such as object-relations theory or some versions of humanistic psychology, which also seem to promise internal harmony if only the environment is right (Frosch, 1987, p. 109). But it never is right, which can make the promise seem spurious and the environ-mentalism a mere mask for as pessimistic a determinism as the grimmer forms of psychoanalysis can offer. RC would seem even more open to this charge, since its concept of what is required for healthy development and of what is pathogenic is so wide. Being lied to, being treated with disrespect, discovering that you live in a society in which you are called on to spend more and more while people starve else-where, that you are being fed toxic foods by those who love you, who feel power-less to do otherwise – all these are hurtful, even abusive experiences. However, RC has an equally wide notion of our capacities to heal and our opportunities to do so, through the process of taking turns offering each other good, non-judgemental attention, through emotional discharge even of the oldest hurts and subsequent insight ('re-evaluation') and change. For our purposes here, what is relevant is how RC manages to have a theory of oppression which is not a deficit model.

For RC, if a group's needs are systematically unmet on the pretext of some supposed characteristic of that group, the group is oppressed. There is not neces-sarily any other group which acts as a particular agent of the oppression, though there may be. Thus parents are oppressed, but not by their children; men are oppressed (by virtue of being treated as expendable in work and war), but not by women, while white people do act as the particular agents of the oppression of black people. Even in these latter cases, oppression is viewed as a function of social structures, not of any inherent vices of the group which gains material benefits. Oppression begins in childhood: children are systematically oppressed by virtue of being treated with lack of respect, even when they are not sexually abused, neglected or used for the parent's or other adult's gratification or consolation. The role of victim is uncomfortable and frightening, so the young one is likely to move into an oppressive or controlling role – especially if such a role is socially sanctioned, as it is for boys. If we had not been systematically hurt as young ones, (while being told we were not hurting and being deprived of the chance to discharge about it) we would never be willing, RC believes, to take up oppressive positions in our turn.

The sequence of brutalization, numbing and repetition of the oppressive experience from the other position is clearly illustrated in British public schools, where boys are (or were) 'systematically tortured and degraded in the most inhumane ways . . . [and] then manipulated in later years into the other end of the pattern, forced to give the same vicious treatment to younger boys in preparation for their "ruling" role' (Jackins, 1983, p. 64). This mechanism is well-known, but RC claims it exists in less obvious ways throughout daily social life and that oppressive social structures depend on and bring about its constant reproduction.

RC's theory of oppression describes how various groups are affected by the material conditions of their social position and the cultural meanings given to it, how their ideas of themselves are constructed from this experience and how it permits them to remain in touch with and to use some aspects of their human potential but bars access to other aspects of it. As in deficit models, RC shows how oppression has a harmful effect on the oppressed. But it also claims that it has an equally harmful psychological effect on the oppressor, even if the latter benefits materially. Human nature is such, and human connection and interdependence such, that it is psychologically hurtful for us to hurt others. Class is the perfect example, relatively neglected by radical therapies as well as by equal opportunities policy-makers. Jackins argues that class structures once had positive aspects 'in the historical settings of their emergence', but now no longer have (Jackins, 1981, p. 469). All class societies, according to him, dehumanize *all* human beings contained within them. At the root of class issues is the patterned feeling of being inferior which is installed in all children, a ready-made template for class meanings and also for racism and sexism (Jackins, 1989, p. 227). The feeling of being superior is merely the 'other end' of the same 'distress recording' – the oppressive role is often more comfortable than that of the oppressed (Jackins, 1978, p. 297). This double-sided foundation narrows the repertoire of likely responses when, throughout life, typical hurtful experiences happen to people in particular class positions. Working-class children, for example, are likely to be told in one way or another that they are stupid. This repeated hurtful experience results in typical patterns (not trusting your own thinking, deferring to the 'clever') which are crucial to the reproduction of the class structure. Middle-class children are more likely to learn that they are privileged, but that their privileges are insecure and may be taken away if they *look* stupid.

Although I have simplified this difference and said next to nothing about the mechanisms through which it is supposed to arise, it is possible to see that this is not a deficit model. To the extent that working-class people are debarred from the confident full use of their intelligence, they are hurt and damaged by the class system. In other respects they may be more 'in touch with their humanness', more able (for example) to notice what is actually going on between people, who is being straightforward and who is pulling rank or being devious. The class system permits *this* sort of intelligence to working class people. Middle-class people may have more access to their intellectual powers, but their use of these tends to be limited to certain types of situation and is often contaminated by a fear of being exposed as incompetent, of loss of privilege, and of loss of the early love current privileges symbolize. This may result in a layer of pretence or pretentiousness, which is itself a hurtful effects of the class system. '*Everybody* is oppressed. *Everybody's* life is ruined by living in an oppressive society, *everybody's*! Even the members of the oppressing classes can be reached intellectually (individually, not as a class, of course) to want to end oppression' (Jackins, 1978, p. 389). Along similar lines the international leader of black people in RC, Barbara Love, tells whites not to speak of 'my racism', but to remember that they never wanted to be separated from people of colour. Oppression, she writes, is characteristically divisive. It not only divides white people from black people, but creates divisions within each group in the process known as 'internalised oppression'. Love urges white people to respect and value each other, as an essential step towards making good relationships with black people (Love, 1994).

RC is open to the criticism commonly levelled at humanistic theories: that it espouses a version of biology-society dualism in which the 'true self', the 'individual', is essentially formed at conception but is distorted and rendered rigid and irrational by society. Although so much causal weight is attributed to the social environment, its role is merely to restrict or enable the spontaneous development of the original 'true self'. There is no articulated understanding that we only live, think and act *through* culture and that RC's particular application of 'a natural process' is the product of a culturally specific moment. However, RC's 'true self' could be understood as a set of potentialities, of human capacities and liabilities, rather than as a finished homunculus. These capacities demand a suitable sociocultural context to be realized, but otherwise remain intact as unmet needs and unused powers. RC's dualistic insistence on the good true self as distinct from 'pseudo-reality' can be seen as a *political* insistence on opposing the view that the restrictions it sees as effects of hurt are in fact the natural frontiers of human development.

Part of RC's project is to build and rebuild human cultures and societies appropriate both to the timeless aspects of human nature and to the material and social conditions that now exist. This involves a judicious sorting through, reassembly and creative reworking of existing cultural materials and social practices:

> All our cultures are composites of useful lore or knowledge and of 'cultural' patterns, and . . . part of our re-emergence consists of examining these cultures and differentiating between their components, respecting and sharing the valuable lore, and rejecting and discharging the patterns . . . we will be left with only our strengths. (Jackins, 1992, p. 34)

A far cry this from postmodernism and likely to draw down the wrath of anthropologists such as Geertz, who argues fiercely against a position in which cultural diversity across space and over time, amounts to a series of expressions, some salubrious, some not, of a settled, underlying reality, the essential nature of man, and anthropology amounts to an attempt to see through the haze of those expressions to the substance of that reality. (Geertz, 1984, p. 272)

Any such attempt to find the essential in human nature must assume that 'culture is icing, biology, cake; that we have no choice as to what we shall hate (hippies? bosses? eggheads? . . . relativists?) that difference is shallow, likeness deep' (Geertz, 1984, p. 268).

From a critical realist point of view, Geertz's revulsion is misplaced. The 'human nature' is shorthand for various causally generative structures and mechanisms (human capacities and psychological structures and processes) which can never be realized or effective outside of culture. It would therefore be absurd to call them 'biological' in the sense of an *opposition* to culture. We could more usefully see both human psychological structures and human social structures as simultaneously made possible and constrained by human physiology (presumably Geertz would grant this?). We can also see them as emerging *from each other* – as establishing each other's conditions of possibility (see Chapter 2, pp. 18–20). This means that there can never be a cultural form which directly expresses the 'substance' of human nature, no 'final' or 'true' culture, for all must express that substance. To say this 'makes difference shallow' is simply to say that human beings are all human. However, RC's project of sorting through cultural products for the more 'salubrious' is itself historically situated and culturally produced, not the gateway to any final harmony and stasis.

Nevertheless, in its rejection of deficit models and view of all humans as oppressed, RC expects its healing process to free the imagination and assist people to identify with all other humans. Among other ways of helping people free themselves from internalized oppression, RC uses the slogan 'claim it, clean it up, throw it out'. Identities connected with oppressive social structures, such as 'working class', 'English', or 'bisexual', need to be claimed (though it may well not be appropriate to do so publicly). The person's significance and goodness (and all the other characteristics of the true self) must be claimed and recognized *from that identity*, which may feel difficult. (For example, a woman may have no difficulty in recognizing that she is intelligent, but find it hard to believe if she focuses on remembering she is also a working-class woman. Working on this will bring healing emotional discharge.)

This is the claiming and 'cleaning up'. When this is done, the label (which is seen as an artefact born of oppression) should become less and less important and eventually the co-counsellor should start work on giving it up. What they are giving up is not female genitals or a certain skin colour, but the internal baggage that has got attached to the social significance of these. Some have experimented with getting co-counsellors to work on being a woman (if a man) or a man (if a woman) or a black person (if white) and so on, seeing everything from that other per~
This is reminiscent of the old joke 'Anyone can be a Jew. You just

chicken soup with knaidlach, potato latkes at Chanukka, read the Talmud, drink four glasses of wine at Pesach, tell Jewish jokes and have a close family life. Apart from that there's only the oppression – and who wants that?' Here RC, in most respects anathema to postmodernism, agrees with it that categories are ultimately arbitrary – although social divisions are material and real.

Another self-help network, CONNECT, began in 1983 running meetings and workshops on the nuclear issue, on feminism, psychohistory and other subjects. CONNECT describes itself as 'interested in linking individual change to political and social change' (leaflet and application form). It is now largely a correspondence group, focusing on discussing circulated papers. RC sees class structures and other forms of oppression as psychologically damaging to perpetrators as well as to victims and as parasitic on the disempowering effects of previous oppression. In one of the 'CONNECT papers' David Wasdell goes even further beyond a deficit model (Wasdell, 1989). In this pamphlet Wasdell embraces what Samuels has called 'the fantasy . . . of providing therapy for the world', where Samuels is not implying that the fantasy is pathological, for 'right now the fantasy of treating the world is empathic with, in tune with the world's desire to be treated, the clamour of the world for therapeutic attention' (Samuels, 1993, p. 29). Wasdell redefines the political activist as a 'social analyst' who can never get free of the fantasies of the analysand, which the analyst must also share. The social analyst must continually struggle against the pressure to collude, from inside themselves as well as from others. Success in pointing out 'the oppressive and repressive dynamics' of 'unwanted unconscious content' inevitably leads to attack:

> As the analyst identifies the common split-off parts of the social psyche and integrates them within his own being, so he becomes identified with those same parts within the social process. Unless there is significant progress in social integration he is subjected to projective identification . . . The analyst becomes 'the enemy' though also 'the saviour'

in what Wasdell terms a process of 'social transference' (1989, p. 3).

Wasdell believes that whole groups re-enact conflicts that affected all, or nearly all, their members in earlier life. The key one of these from the point of view of understanding modern societies is the foetal experience of malnutrition when the placenta fails during birth. For Wasdell, war and other forms of destruction and religion and other attempts at reachieving unity are the result of fixations at the level of pre-birth:

> Because we are fixated at placental failure, we assume the environment is an unlimited source. But in fact the earth is not an infinitely resourceful womb . . . nor an unlimited sink . . . Foetal assumptions persist because the fixation was so intense. Reality can only be faced and acted on, if the defences and consequent fantasies are deconstructed. (Collingwood, 1992, p. 3)

As always with monocausal approaches, a great variety of phenomena become unintelligible because the single posited cause cannot explain their differences and their development. In his critique of Wasdell, Collingwood attempts to give capitalism its specificity and distinctiveness by integrating Wasdell's approach with Marxism. For our purposes what is important is that here is another radical theory, a highly eclectic one drawing on Klein, Grof, Lake and Gestalt, which sees our present societies as psychologically damaging to *all*. 'Previously medicine has seen sickness as deviation from the norm. Likewise psychanalysis. Today we face the psychopathology of the norm iself. Health depends on deviation from it ... our civilisation is unconsciously shaped and is in danger of termination' (Collingwood, 1992, p. 4).

Conclusion

This chapter has scanned four sorts of radical therapy and the theories they have given rise to. All would give roughly similar answers to our two questions. In answer to the first question: 'What is psychological health? Does it involve social criticism and political action?' they would reply that psychological health must involve a grasp on social reality, including the nature and outrageousness of oppressive social relations and the real value of self and others in the teeth of social invalidation. To get such an understanding and to hold on to it necessarily means sticking up for oneself and others and finding ways of taking action against oppression. These theories may completely disagree about what oppressive structures exist, who should act and how. To the extent that they hold to a 'deficit model' their analysis of oppressive structures arguably fails and remains stuck at the perspective of oppression as 'normal'.

In answer to the second question: 'What is the relationship between psychic structures and social structures?', all radicals would agree that these are causally interlinked, so that each contributes to the reproduction of the other. But here 'specialist' theories, like feminist therapy or transcultural therapy, are at an advantage. If women, or black people, have been robbed of some of their human potential, we have at least examplars of other groups who have not been deprived in just this way. We have some idea of what we want back. This approach threatens to lead to a deficit model, but need not. We can envision for ourselves the strengths socially available to other groups, while still recognizing and avoiding their own limitations. Indeed, if we see everyone as damaged and unable to free themselves from the compromising baggage of early hurts, there is nowhere to stand in order to exercise transformative power.

The theories discussed above addressed inequalities associated with 'race' and ethnicity, gender and class. Of those considered, only the CONNECT material referred directly to the effects of our present social structures on the planet we inhabit. But ecological destruction is mediated through all these other power relations, which are all relevant to the development of strategies against ecological destruction. The requirement of the economic South for 'development' is the historical legacy of imperialist relations and colonialism, as well as present-day economic domination through global capitalism and transnational corporations. Environmental destruction is resulting from the structural adjustment programmes imposed on debtor countries by the World Bank. And within rich countries, toxic waste and environmental risk is unevenly distributed along lines of 'race' and class. Eco-feminists point out that the major institutions producing environmental degradation – governments, their militaries and transnationals – are by and large controlled by men and dominated by masculine culture (Seager, 1993, p. 5). The perpetrators on one dimension are among the victims on others. Radicals who address specific forms of oppression offer an important contribution to green strategies, but the most hopeful theories may well be those which, while rejecting health-as-normal-functioning, offer their 'therapy for the world' to all.

Chapter 9

Conclusion: If humanly possible

Four necessary conditions for radical change

Chapter 2 argued that to understand the scope of human agency and its ecopolitical implications, we need to theorize human psychological nature, especially the relationship between psychological and social structures and the notion of health. Chapter 3 looked at discourses of health, a key form taken by such theorizing. In particular, it concluded that there is a contradiction between notions of health-as-normal-functioning and the notions of positive health which can found social criticism. This distinction is closely related to the distinction made in Chapter 2 between the role of agents as reproducing social structures and their role as transforming them. I argued that transformative action has to be deliberate and involves an articulated rupture with 'business as usual' and a corresponding rejection of everyday conformist notions of health. I described four characteristics of human nature which have to be the case for radical social change to be possible, including the change to an ecologically sustainable society. These are necessary but obviously not sufficient for such a radical transformation, which also depends on conditions in the rest of the world. Yet the conditions affecting agency may seem daunting enough.

The 'four conditions' were:

1   Human beings have to be capable of developing *the will to change* to ecologically sustainable societies in large numbers – and human motivations have to be able to take this form now, in our present societies.
2   Agents of change, individual and collective, have to be capable of *awareness of reality* in relation to environmental threat and its causes. This has to be possible now, in our present societies. We must not only know, but be able to take in and act on the knowledge.
3   *Movements* have to be built which incorporate and encourage such motivation and such thinking, without self-sabotage. This means they have to be, or to become, capable of minimizing and dealing with internal attacks and splits.

4   The envisioned new societies must be ones in which human beings are capable of living, i.e. they must be *humanly sustainable*.

Now that we have reviewed the views of a range of psychotherapeutic theories on human nature, psychological health and on the relationship between psychological and social structures, it is useful to sum up their contributions in terms of these four conditions. This provides us with no guide as to their relative truth. It is notoriously hard to judge the truth value of theories at such a level of abstraction, most of which link with the world mainly through clinical practice. Bock assumes that human nature theories always lack empirical bite and that we should decide between these accounts in terms of how we want to be, making an ethical choice between these competing narratives (Bock, 1994, p. 114). In relation to agency, he argues that we should choose an 'open' human nature mythology which stresses human potential and human responsibility:

> Humans, as Picodella Mirandola told us, should regard themselves as capable of anything. We should take that as a moral premise. We should decide we are like that. (ibid.)

In fact there *are* other ways of judging between theories of human nature. How comprehensive an account does the theory offer of the phenomena it addresses? How effective is it as a guide to practice? Are there other ways of accounting for the phenomena, including those resulting from putting this theory into practice? How internally consistent is the theory? How does it relate to other, highly valued and useful theories? For example, I suggested in Chapter 5 that Klein's notion of envy as innate is implausible in terms of the theory of evolution. If truth were no more than use value, this would hardly be an objection. But usefulness is usually an indication of a degree of adequacy in describing the world. Pragmatic and ethical considerations certainly inform our theoretical choices, but these are grounded in reality. Grounded, rather than founded. If these are foundations, they are partial and shifting. But in this area, partial (that is, ordinary) knowledge, work in progress, is very welcome. There is sometimes convergence between these usually incompatible perspectives (when they address the same field of phenomena) which can be recognized with interest as mutually reinforcing, without falling into a promiscuous eclecticism.

The ecopolitics of rival psychologies

What light, then, can our theories cast on the 'four conditions'? I shall leave Lacan out, for I think Chapter 6 demonstrated his antipathy to this whole approach and his irrelevance to it.

Freud and ego-psychology

Freud's late theory and its more direct descendants would certainly see human beings as capable of such motivation and such awareness, although not likely to realize this potential in great numbers.

(1) the will to change

The main source of the will to build a more rational society is the sublimation of erotic urges. Want and distress militate against such sublimation on a wide scale. However, religion, which is also fuelled by modified libido, need not be deterred by social injustice, so an ecological movement with the wish-fulfilment characteristics of a religion could become popular.

(2) awareness of reality

However, the very characteristics that permit popularity are obstacles to flexible rational thinking and awareness of reality.

The long term trend of civilization, Freud hoped, was towards greater synthesis and rationality, including an extension of our moral communities. But even if that extension could be envisaged as leading to anything like ecological consciousness, it would be a very slow process. Freudian theory, then, supports reformist environmentalism, rather than deep ecology, radical green socialism or anarchism. Since relatively few are likely to achieve the psychological health required to invest in realistic and appropriate political change, leadership will be required and institutional ways of encouraging others. Freud provides us with a way of understanding why and in what way human beings are irrational – that consumer goods are substitutes for the fulfilment of early sexual wishes, and so on.

(3) movements

As for green movements, Freudian theory offers a theory of leadership and a vocabulary invaluable to understanding – and perhaps mitigating – processes of scapegoating, splitting and exclusion, but without any hope of preventing or finally overcoming these.

(4)   human social possibilities

We can assume Freud's answer to the question of whether human beings are capable of building and maintaining a just, ecologically sustainable society, would be much like his view on the possibility of eliminating war: a good idea, but vulnerable to constant sabotage from the internal springs of aggression and destruction. So from a Freudian viewpoint, I suspect a benevolent authoritarian environmentalism, limiting but still relying on the market, would be the most hopeful way forward.

Klein and the Kleinians

(1)   will to change

In practice Kleinians, like Freudians, tend to be suspicious of 'extremism', since wherever there is a hated enemy there must be processes of projection and consequent unawareness. But in theory human beings are certainly capable of developing the will to social change, based on impulses towards reparation. They are unlikely to do so consistently or in large numbers, though, because present consumerist societies mass-produce motivations that draw so effectively on human greed, aggression and envy. We are not happy like this, it is true, but unhappiness and the addictions that mask it are eminently ordinary.

(2)   awareness of reality

Hoggett, using post-Kleinian theory, discusses the 'apparently mad behaviour undertaken by apparently normal individuals' in terms of the requirement of the social medium, the prospective container, that we share *its* 'state of mind' (1992, p. 74). A social context in which 'our own better knowledge proves difficult to bear ... tends to elicit from people an orientation to the world which is neither psychotic denial nor neurotic acceptance but ... on the borderline of the two' (1992, p. 77). The caring, flattering, secretly threatening and openly reassuring voices of the media, terrify and enfold us in a single paragraph or image. The facts about the ozone hole are known, but simply cannot be taken in, and such taking in is a precondition for action. Awareness of reality has constantly to be struggled for when that reality is so anxiety-provoking.

(3) movements

Could social movements be built which allowed this to be done and which were genuinely reparative? It may well be so. Hoggett argues that the psychoanalytic tradition has been too wary of groups and has tended to forget the virtues of grandiosity (1992, p. 148). He suggests the 'combined parent figure (strong but gentle)' as a model for the agency 'most capable of leading social movements in an effective struggle against the external establishment' (1992, p. 96). The 'Revolutionary Work Group' needs no formal discipline; its members are bound by their collective desire and imagination. Its task is to create a culture which can contain fears of betrayal, disillusionment and so on, so that it need not have recourse 'to a formal establishment' – rules, cards and suchlike rigidities – and which can recognize this as a danger (1992, p. 158). Its practice needs to be a 'playful and interrogative process of reality-testing' (Hoggett draws on Winnicott here) which explores the 'give' in existing power relations and the scope of agency (1992, p. 155). It needs to fulfil its members' potentials, to stretch, engage and amuse them.

(4) human social possibilities

Can we live in better societies, or are we obliged to spoil the good? As we have seen, Kleinian theory does not believe in possible social perfection. Splitting processes, destructive urges, greed are here to stay, but need not take the form of destroying the very medium of life. They could undoubtedly be minimized by aware social policies and reflective practices, though it is unclear just what political forms these might take. Although Hoggett praises a libertarianism which avoids fixity, I suspect Rustin's social-democratic welfare society would be a more likely form for Kleinian environmentalism.

Humanistic psychologies

Humanistic psychologists are closest to ecopolitical groupings in their philosophy and have actually inspired various organizational practices. For them, as for many object-relations theorists, it is at least theoretically possible for individuals and society to be in harmony. Humans *can* produce institutions which are in tune with our cooperative nature and from this, benign circles can spiral outwards.

(1) will to change

The will to change is present in all humans, merely dormant. Oppression and want certainly make it harder to tap (as Maslow outlined in his theory of need). This should incline humanistic theorists more to social ecology or similar positions linking ecology and social justice. But some simply ignore such supposed structural obstacles to insight and assume that a dormant intuition can be awoken in anyone, however situated, through education, leadership, inspiration and spiritual experiences.

(2) awareness of reality

Compared with psychoanalysis, humanistic psychologies have a more rationalistic view of the awareness of reality, more faith in the conscious mind and especially in the power of education, consciousness-raising and experience-sharing – and in experience generally.

(3) movements

Movements have to be built which offer such consciousness-raising and support and in which people can give each other something like the 'unconditional positive regard' and good listening which Rogers believes is such a strong mutative factor. Those trained in humanistic psychology have ways of doing things which can, they believe, bring this about. These include minimizing hierarchy by rotating chairs and other democratic practices, treating all with respect by inviting everyone to speak and to contribute to the agenda, ensuring meetings are not dominated by habitual talkers and so on. However, the fringe workshop on 'hugging' at one British Green Party conference brought some unwelcome media attention.

(4) human social possibilities

Humanistic psychologies are confident that they know how to bring about cultures (and presumably also economic structures) which are consonant with human nature in a way our present ones are not. Human disconnection from nature is part of a general malaise, so political action towards a more rational society should, in the medium and long term, make us feel better and provide its own reinforcing motivation.

Radicals

For radicals who 'specialize' in the psychological effects of particular sorts of oppression, it seems clear that unless these are addressed, the still-oppressed will be unable to ignore their present situation and take action on the ecological front alone.

(1)   will to change

The will to change can only be reached by addressing present, differentiated sources of suffering. These can neither be reduced to a wider concern, nor postponed.

(2)   awareness of reality

Oppression militates against awareness of many aspect of social reality, while at the same time making the oppressed super-sensitive to some of the detailed mechanisms through which their mistreatment takes place. To the extent that invalidating messages enter the process of the construction of subjectivity, people *have* to address their own oppression as members of whichever groups, before they can realistically take on wider issues. Indeed, the recognition and naming of oppressive social relations is part of the awareness of reality, essential to realistic ecopolitics. Ecological movements that hardly include women, that have no specific understanding of how women's position affects and is affected by environmental degradation, are seriously limiting the power of their analyses – as well as their ability to recruit women to their ranks.

The radical suggestion that specific oppressions have to be addressed before wider ecological issues can be taken on (Bookchin, 1995, p. 122) is reminiscent of Maslow's hierarchy of needs and we saw that for Maslow the B-cognizers seemed to be fairly privileged (Maslow, 1973, p. 328). I shall discuss in the last section of this chapter the seeming implication of all deficit models, that the more privileged are inevitably healthier and more effective ecopolitical agents and reconsider there the other radical position that being the agent of oppression also gravely interferes with awareness of inner and outer reality.

(3)   movements

Here, let us simply note that for radicals, effective ecological movements *must* also address social justice issues, or will remain very limited in their social basis.

In the US, for example, 'some communities are routinely poisoned while the government looks the other way' or, worse, cynically plans to dump toxic wastes in socially vulnerable poor neighbourhoods inhabited mainly by people of colour (Bullard, 1994, p. 254). Few mainstream environmental groups:

> have actively involved themselves in environmental conflicts involving communities of color. Because of this, it's unlikely that we will see a mass influx of people of color into the national environmental groups . . . A continuing growth in their own grassroots organisations is more likely. (1994, p. 262)

However, if mainstream movements can (as is increasingly happening) openly recognize and oppose environmental racism, this would itself be a healing move.

Radicals come from so many backgrounds that it is hard to generalize about (3) and (4). We could say as regards (3) that radicals may be more willing than practising professional psychotherapists openly to reject everyday notions of health. This rejection *could* (but need not) help them devise new ways of organizing which actively counteract splitting and scapegoating tendencies.

(4) human social possibilities

Dorothy Rowe can serve as an example of radical thinking here. In her book *Living with the Bomb*, she explores how fears about nuclear war are usually denied (along with other painful memories and fears) in a costly process that 'pushes us further and further away from reality, both our external and internal reality' and makes us behave stupidly and inappropriately (Rowe, 1985, p. 46). The book's subtitle is 'Can we live without enemies?' and its concluding chapter outlines the psychological preconditions of lasting peace. International understanding and forgiveness, according to Rowe, requires:

1 Seeing the Stranger (our enemy) as person, not object;
2 Separating the hurtful act from the actor;
3 Accepting that our knowledge, our viewpoint, is partial;
4 Creating a shared language, seeing the other's point of view;
5 Understanding that the Stranger is afraid of us, too;
6 Accepting our own and others' anger;
7 Being prepared to forgive.

Much of her argument can be applied, *mutatis mutandis*, to the search for ecological sustainability, given the enormous international redistribution that would be required. She herself is unsure about our human capacity to live without enemies. But, like other radicals, when asked whether ecologically sustainable societies would be possible for humans to live in, she might reply that our *present* societies aren't humanly possible and are daily becoming less so.

Embryonic green psychologies

If within each psychology lies an embryonic ecopolitics, what are the more or less developed psychologies of different green positions?

Environmentalism

Let us look first at the range most readily described in terms of what it is *not*: environmentalism, or green reformism. 'Shallow ecology' in terms of Arne Naess's (1955c) dichotomy 'argues for a managerial approach to environmental problems, secure in the belief that they can be solved without fundamental changes in present values or patterns of production or consumption' (Dobson, 1995, p. 1). However, this definition makes it sound rather *too* shallow. Even if environmentalists believe that existing institutions (including nation States, the market and the UN) can be reformed to halt or limit environmental destruction and allow repair, this remains an awesome task. Recycling on a hitherto unimagined scale, taxation of pollution, changes in transport systems and in consumption, the redistribution of income from rich to poor countries – this is the terrain of the Brundtland report as well as of concrete policies of many green parties and organizations. For believers, the 'security' Dobson mentions is tempered by the belief that this option is on offer for a limited time only.

(1) and (2) will to change, awareness of reality

Even if it looks 'shallow' in comparison with 'deep' ecology, a thorough-going environmentalism is incompatible with health-as-normal-functioning. Just because they do *not* pathologize all our current structures of consumption and production, environmentalists are challenged to explain their fellow-citizens' apparent apathy and myopia, their lack of awareness of reality (2) and hence of will to change (1). What's wrong with them? Do they not know and therefore appear not to care? This was an early belief in green movements, which has lost its claim to plausibility. Do they know, but not care anyway? Or do they know a little, but not know what to do and therefore prefer not to know more and merely appear not to care? Environmentalism veers between these positions, usually taking a basic rationalist view of human motivation, sometimes modified with the view that despair, fear and power-lessness are widespread and disabling and best overcome by encouraging people to adopt and save a tree rather than by telling them how many trees fall for ever every time they exhale.

In general, for environmentalism (1) people act according to their material inter-ests, modified by love for those closest to them and commitment to a few aesthetic and moral values. The structures in which we live *can* corrupt. But persuasion, encouragement and example can enable people to take a wider and longer term view of their interests and to extend their moral communities beyond themselves and their immediate kin to wider family, neighbourhood, colleagues, nation and even (in a weaker way) potentially to humankind itself.

(3)   movements

The movements that have to exert this persuasive influence are mostly on tradi-tional lines of electoral parties and pressure groups, since the key actors are gov-ernments, transnational corporations and intergovernmental organizations, but there is some contested influence of humanistic and radical ways of organizing.

(4)   human social possibilities

As for the societies to be built, we already know that humans can live in them, since their general form of relatively strong central authorities combined with plural checks and balances is not unlike what we have now. Just greener.

Social ecology

Bookchin's 'social ecology' represents an important strand of green libertarianism. Bookchin believes that what is distinctive about humans is precisely our capacity to think, to innovate and to change the environment (1995, p. 17). This change need not be domination and destruction: that it has become so is the result of capitalism (rather than of technology or of industrialism *per se*) (Bookchin, 1995, p. 153). Were we animals like any others, as deep ecologists would have it, there could be no harm in our overrunning the planet and destroying other species. It is precisely because of our specifically *human* ethical sensibilities and power of choice that we must not continue to do so. We are not too civilized, as deep ecologists would have it, but 'not civilised enough' (1995, p. 235). Our animal nature is conservative and rigid. As we build societies based on our capacity to reason, we become increasingly human, increasingly ourselves: 'to become human is to become rational and imaginative, thoughtful and visionary, in rectifying the ills of the present society' (Bookchin, 1995, p. 32).

Bookchin is no Freudian, but if Freud were an environmentalist today he might well be attracted to aspects of social ecology. Here are his own evolutionary beliefs, his own rationalism, his own dislike of mysticism and reverence for science and an anthropology that could almost step out of *The Future of an Illusion*, without the gloom of *Civilisation and its Discontents*. Like Freud, Bookchin sees reason as hindered by emotion; that is why he sees no positive aspects to deep ecological attempts at general therapy. Capitalism is inherently mystificatory. We have simply mistaken our own interests under the sway of its ideology or been too pressurized by want and oppression to be able to think about ecology. Social justice will release our human psychological capacities to reason. Bookchin combines the élitism of an Adorno with the optimism of the early Enlightenment that he so impressively defends:

> Either humanity is merely an animal species, perhaps more destructive than most, subject to blind and overwhelming 'forces of Nature' ... or it is a remarkable *transformative* agent that has produced ... a radical new evolutionary pathway of unequalled creativity and promise in giving meaning to the planet ... [there *is* a need] for a new sensibility – one that highly values animals, forests and ecological diversity – as *only* human beings can. (Bookchin, 1995, p. 235)

(1) will to change

Human beings can develop the will to change by becoming free from capitalist mystification and can be ethically motivated (Bookchin rejects the sociobiological reduction of altruism to 'selfishness').

(2) awareness of reality

Psychological health certainly involves the awareness of reality for Bookchin, but he is not particularly interested in *inner* reality, nor does he pay any attention to the idea that humans are numb or despairing rather than mystified and oppressed.

(3) movements

Movements can and must be built which involve participatory democracy and accountability – the appeal to reason is again the main tool for this process.

(4) human social possibilities

As for human beings' capacity to live in the envisioned new society, that will not be a problem since it is far more consonant with our real nature than destructive capitalism. As Bookchin's politics represent a vigorous defence of Enlightenment ideals, his psychology is a firm no-nonsense return to the unitary subject.

It would be unfair to suggest that all other anarchist, libertarian and socialist greens share Bookchin's psychological outlook, though many do. His work is valuable in its intelligent and consistent articulation of an uncompromising position. For others, rationalism is not enough. Capitalist consumerism produces the very motivations that reproduce it in a vicious circle that needs imaginative interruption. Socially produced emotional hurts can wreck transformative social movements unless preventive measures are taken and traditional hierarchical organizations cannot prepare us for a fully participatory society. Thus, for example, the English Green Party has an Emotional Needs Working Group. Two of its members explain:

> political activity and personal development need to happen simultaneously. Neither can solve the ecological crisis without the other ... [There is a] close connection between emotional deprivation, environmental destruction and social oppression. Unresolved emotional conflict can emerge as negative behaviour. Anatagonising fellow-activists does nothing to bring the arms trade to an end, nor does it create the goodwill necessary for the development and implementation of effective policies. (Christian and Isserlis, 1993, p. 4)

Deep ecology

Deep ecology, though, tends to go further. True, some ecocentrics advocate the most traditional and conservative of organizational forms and their implicit psychologies see human nature as inherently hierarchical – and patriarchal. For others, hierarchy and the urge to domination both stem from a widespread pathology which cannot be attributed to capitalist mystification alone. Its effects are to interfere with thinking and awareness of reality (for example, in the widespread refusal to recognize limits to growth) and in a failure of perception: a pathological inability to notice our deep connectedness, as humans, with all other life forms and the planet itself.

> Whatever the cultural elaboration of the human, its basic physiological as well as psychic nourishment and support came from the surrounding natural environment. In the beginning, human society was integrated with ... the larger earth community, composed of all the geological as well as biological and human elements. Just how long this primordial harmony endured we do not know. (Berry, 1995, p. 9)

Nor what, we might add, you could possibly mean by it.

Be that as it may, many deep ecologists believe that the loss of an original state of harmony with the natural world has resulted in a deep, planet-wide cultural pathology which affects all humans. We are suffering from post-traumatic stress disorder, shown in such symptoms as 'inappropriate bursts of anger, psychic numbing, constriction of emotions [and] loss of a sense of control over our destiny' (Glendenning, 1995, p. 37). We react by turning to addictions: to psychotropic drugs, food, TV and the like, attempting in vain to satisfy our primary needs through secondary sources. As the wildernesses shrink, we continue to lose touch with the wildness within ourselves (Snyder, 1995, p. 49). 'A kind of madness arises from the prevailing nature-conquering, nature-hating and self-and-world denial' (Shepard, 1995, p. 139).

Capra suggests that our civilization is 'emotionally immature' (1995, p. 29). 'With maturity, human beings will experience joy when another life form experiences joy, and sorrow when other life forms experience sorrow' (ibid.). The 'oceanic feeling' that Freud saw as a regression to the state of infancy before the establishment of clear ego boundaries (1961c, p. 59) is understood by deep ecologists as a prefigurative experience of a more mature (and wholly realistic) notion of the self. Naess (1995c), for instance, argues that if the social self, the self in relationship, is considered more mature than the egoistic self (as it is in ego-psychology), the 'ecological self' should be recognized as another step to psychological maturity.

We can recognize, in the half-mature state that passes for normal moral functioning, that ecological devastation harms us humans directly. But we are also capable of extending our identifications to transcend our individual physical and species boundaries and include fleas, plants, even landscapes and rivers. Such an extension realizes inherent human potentialities. Naess argues that the places we are rooted in, the localities and the planet itself, are not *external* to us. They are, in a sense, part of us, since we are changed by their destruction. Naess encourages us to emphasize:

> the conditions under which we most naturally widen and deepen the 'self'. With a sufficiently wide and deep 'self', *ego* and *alter* as opposites are, stage by stage, eliminated . . . Now is the time . . . [for] a deepening iden-tification with all life forms and the greater units: the ecosystems and Gaia, the fabulous old planet of ours. (Naess, 1995c, p. 235)

If we widen the self in this way, the loss of species becomes an arguably greater tragedy than human suffering.

Samuels suggests that despite the *real* danger of apocalypse, certain fantasies of it 'are the deepest sign of a self-punishing contempt for ourselves. Perhaps many people think we deserve to perish like this' (1993, p. 15). He sees ecologism as split between those who project all blame on to others (capitalism, men, developed nations, etc.) and those who, blaming humans including themselves, attempt 'to make reparation and repentance over-literally – by making it up to the entire planet' (ibid.). Misanthropy and self-punishing rejection of *any* desire to use technology to improve human lives are certainly significant strands in deep ecology. But perhaps those who think of human beings as deeply lost, rather than wicked, are less vulnerable to these ugly byproducts of the 'widening of the self'.

Joanna Macy is an influential ecological activist who runs workshops on despair and empowerment. In *World as Lover, World as Self* she argues from this experience that the loss of 'the certainty that we have a future . . . felt at some level of consciousness by everyone, regardless of political orientation, is the pivotal psychological reality of our time' (1991, p. 5). According to Macy, despair 'lurks subliminally beneath the tenor of life-as-usual' (cf. health-as-normal-functioning). Yet this emotion is culturally taboo and 'the refusal to feel takes a heavy toll' on our capacity for joy, our perception and our ability to think, for we process out anxiety-provoking data, which is feedback we urgently need in order to take intelligent, effective action (1991, p. 15). 'The distance between our inklings of apocalypse and the tenor of business-as-usual is so great that . . . we tend to imagine that it is we, not the society, who are insane' (1991, p. 19). Psychotherapists are little use because they tend, in reductionist mode, to believe it impossible that present threats to the collective welfare should so distress us.

Macy holds the deep ecological view, consonant with some versions of humanistic psychology, with RC and with versions of analytical psychology, that humans are inherently deeply interconnected. Our social despair is, then, completely valid and needs no reduction for its explanation. This despair can be worked through, Macy claims, if it is acknowledged and listened to. Since creative thinking and effective political action can arise out of such work, it needs to be incorporated in ecological social movements. Macy welcomes the notion of 'the greening of the self', the 'widening' proposed by Naess and others, which is scorned by Bookchin and other materialists for its dependence on untestable 'intuitions' and its anthropomorphism. For him, the extension of the self to its ecological surroundings is not self-realization but its opposite – the loss of identity and differentiation, with a corresponding loss of agency.

In contrast, for Macy the self is always a metaphor, a drawing of boundaries that can well be redrawn elsewhere. Morality is a human capacity made necessary by separateness. How much more valuable to the project of healing the planet is identity:

> I don't need to say 'Oh, don't saw off your leg. That would be an act of violence.' It wouldn't occur to me because your leg is part of your body. Well, so are the trees in the Amazon rain forest. They are our external lungs . . . we are beginning to realise that the world is our body. (Macy, 1991, p. 192)

(1) will to change

In the embryonic psychology of deep ecology, the will to change can be fuelled by the gradual realization and diagnosis of our own individual versions of the general malaise. The 'greening of the self' brings its own healing and its own satisfaction.

(2) awareness of reality

Rational argument cannot effect such an insight: awareness of reality is not a matter of scanning lists of facts, but of letting go the defences against emotional (and spiritual) awareness. Experience is only a source of knowledge once this is done, but when the shift *does* take place, intuition and empathy become important resources.

(3) movements

Movements must be built which permit the emotional healing necessary, which are spiritually rich, allowing people to develop their true human potential: 'self-realisation' and 'the ecological self'.

(4) human social possibilities

Certainly humans will be psychologically capable of living in an ecologically sustainable society. Culturally and materially, though, their lives will be very different. And there will need to be far fewer of them.

Ecofeminism

To move from deep ecology to ecofeminism is a short step but a startling change of perspective. Ecofeminists are generally thought of as straightforward essentialists who see women as 'naturally' closer to nature, as having, by virtue of wombs, feeding breasts and monthly cycles, a quite different psychology from men. Mellor distinguishes these 'affinity' ecofeminists from the 'social' ecofeminists who also see gender differences as implicated in environmental destruction, but view them as socially constructed (1992, p. 61). Dobson makes a similar distinction between 'difference' and 'deconstructive' ecofeminism (1995, p. 193). For the first group, women and men are inherently psychologically different. Women are in tune with life, men with domination and death. The following quotation serves to represent this position:

> Nothing links the human animal and nature so profoundly as women's reproductive system which enables her to share the experience of bringing

forth and nourishing life with the rest of the world. *Whether or not she personally experiences biological mothering*, it is in this that woman is most truly a child of nature and in this . . . lies the wellspring of her strength. (Collard, 1988)

In fact, just as deep ecologists are no longer (publicly at least) misanthropic, thorough-going affinity ecofeminists are nowhere to be found. Even Collard and others who sometimes describe men's and women's psychology as inherently opposed, in other contexts attribute this opposition to cultural forces such as the long-ago overthrow of matriarchy and the present-day sexual division of labour. All, in this sense, are 'social' ecofeminists, but some see men's women-and-nature-hating tendencies as the product of millennia while others see them as having shallower roots: 'groomed since early childhood to become the enactors of patriarchy, they began life in the arms of women and, as little boys . . . were thrilled at the sight of a nest of baby birds . . . or ecstatic with freshly fallen snow' (Plant, 1989, p. 3). All agree that as things are, dominant human culture and psychology have become split between feminine and masculine virtues and principles – reason versus intuition (or emotion), mind versus body, human versus animal, male versus female, nurturance versus domination, etc.

The most useful distinction to be drawn within ecofeminism is between those whose notion of social change relies on the *reversal* of these dualisms, making the hidden underside the new ruling principle, and those who believe they feed off each other and must instead be completely deconstructed. The following are expressions of the first strategic perspective: 'When birth becomes our underlying metaphor . . . the world shifts' (Starhawk, 1989, p. 175) and 'the recovery of the female principle allows a redefinition of growth and productivity as categories linked to the production, not the destruction, of life' (Shiva, 1989, p. 90). In contrast: 'Neither the present understanding of what is female or male is an adequate characterisation of what it is to be human . . . both genders are fraught with pathological behaviours' (Plant, 1989, p. 3). Ecofeminists see such deconstruction as also crucial to the struggle against colonization: 'Increasingly the project of expelling the master from human culture and the project of recognising and changing the colonising politics of western relations to other earth nations converge, and increasingly too both these projects converge with the project of survival' (Plumwood, 1993, p. 195).

(1) will to change

For both currents (which indeed overlap) the will to change comes primarily from women, who are more attuned to nature and will therefore care more about its destruction. But men, too, are capable of suffering from their greater and older disconnection and seeking change as a result.

(2) awareness of reality

Women are the primary agents of change because of their greater awareness of reality, inner and outer. Even under the conditions of a destructive patriarchal capitalism, women's experience of biological as opposed to capitalist time (Mellor, 1992, pp. 256–62), of caring and nurturing, constitutes a rich source of knowledge, a resource for social reconstruction.

(3) movements

Ecological movements need female leadership and when that cannot be achieved women need to organize separately. In the male-dominated eco-establishment the wish to influence decision-makers by being 'reasonable' simply reinforces old dualisms and conventional political agendas (Seager, 1993, p. 187), while Earth First! and other deep ecology groups vary from positive misogyny to mere ignorance and indifference towards gender issues (1993, p. 229). Women's experience, women's values, women's openness to emotion must be used as a resource and integrated into green political practice. Only movements which prefigure the desired end can be effective means towards it. Ecological movements must be non-hierarchical and participatory, drawing on the virtues that have been allotted to women without accepting the restrictions. They will incorporate ritual and symbolism and will themselves be healing for both women and men.

(4) human social possibilities

What the new societies will be like is fairly unclear, as it is for much deep ecology. But certainly they will involve participatory democracy and will be non-patriarchal and non-exploitative societies which respect the natural world. The clear message of ecofeminism is that women would flourish in such societies; there is some disagreement about whether this is also true for men.

Conclusion

Can we humans change our social world so as to ensure human social survival, creating ways of social being which no longer destroy the ecosystems that support us? In answering these questions in my own voice, I draw largely on the radical thinking described in the previous chapter. My exposition will be relatively unsubstantiated, representing a beginning as much as an end.

As the radicals argue, environmental destruction is not the unmediated expression of inbuilt greed and/or aggression, but the result of rapacious socioeconomic systems. Undoubtedly the emotions of greed and aggression and their expression in legitimated social practices are vital to system reproduction. These emotions are part of our human potential, or we could not have them. But this part of our potential is made actual, minute by minute, by structurally determined mistreatment and failure to meet the needs of human beings. As the radicals argue, we respond to fear and abuse, ancient or present, by seeking comfort and distraction in commodities (symbols of love) or by envious or angry attacks on people and institutions which symbolize (and sometimes actually are) the perpetrators or the beneficiaries of our mistreatment.

The intellectual work, amounting to considerable research, necessary to unpick the mechanisms involved in all this is discouraged by denial and by what Hoggett terms the 'institutionalisation of shallowness', in which questions of values – questions of life and death – become split off from normal functioning (1992, p. 104). Although I cannot accept either deep ecology or ecofeminism, I want to offer a brief defence of the view both perspectives share: that we *all* fall short of health.

Is the idea of general psychological ill-health meaningless – rather like the claim that we are *all* and for always alienated or subjected? There is certainly a sense in which, if positive health is a function of human pro-social capacities, we must always fall short of it. I mean something more specific. Maslow's work on the relatively healthy, on human thriving, was held back by his unaware classism (1973, p. 328), but the project itself was valid. We do have evidence of the difference between human psychological suffering and human thriving. Criteria for the latter would arguably include an enhanced capacity for clear thinking, an awareness of reality and the ability to bring about desired environmental change. But these criteria are insufficient, since they could be subsumed under instrumental rationality and they fail to indicate what are appropriate, healthy values. What environmental change is it *healthy* to desire?

In *Feminism and the Mastery of Nature* Plumwood rejects the Kantian ethical framework and its use of the reason/emotion dichotomy to deny action based on particular care and attachment to the status of moral action (1993, p. 167). She argues against the idea of human nature as egoistic and the reductionist notion of self-interest as necessarily excluding reference to the welfare of others. A mother:

> wants health and happiness *for* the child for its sake, as well as for her own. Such intrinsic or essential relationships are not confined to the private sphere, and the sense of loss and despair brought about in most of us by the future prospect of a devastated natural and social environment cannot be explained in terms of isolable individual interests. (Plumwood, 1993, p. 154)

The account of the self as 'a self-contained rational maximiser denies the social and connected nature of the self, which could function in the way the fiction implies for only very limited areas of life' (1993, p. 152). On the other hand, the deep ecological extended self denies difference and incorporates the other into the self, an extreme form of colonization.

If I *am* the mountain whose interests I claim to defend, how can its needs be distinguished from my own? 'The question of just whose response counts for both of us has important political implications' (1993, p. 178). Citing Jessica Benjamin, Plumwood defends a relational account of the self as distinct from others yet 'formed by, bound to and in interaction with . . . [them] through a rich set of relationships which are essential to . . . his or her projects' (1993, p. 156). This avoids the pretence that our care for other species and aspects of the natural world are, or should be, homogenous or egalitarian. On this basis we can care about ourselves, our nearest and dearest and (in certain conditions) can realistically but unevenly extend our concern to those other connected entities, *for their own sakes*: humanity as a whole, including unborn generations and the diversity and complexity of life on the planet.

Plumwood's relational account of the self and the view of ecological self-hood she builds on it are more compatible with the psychologies discussed in this book than either the instrumentalist or the deep ecological views of the self. This is not to deny that people can conceptualize themselves in these other ways and act accordingly. Can we say, though, that the relational self is *healthier*? I think that we can do so in a preliminary way, because both other notions of selfhood are, indeed, fictions which can only be put into practice partially and by denying reality. We really are dependent on and connected with other humans and with the ecosystems we live in. We really are distinct and differentiated from these despite our connection. One criterion for health must be that it is pro-survival *in the long term* and fictions can only have a short-term pragmatic value.

For health-as-normal-functioning, however, the instrumental self has considerable pragmatic value. Even if in family and private life people know themselves to be embedded in many sets of relationships which enter into their projects and interests, the social structures we inhabit almost force instrumentality on us as a defensive measure. When we pass beggars, when we see disasters on the news, when we hear of or witness cruelty or destruction, even though our internal understanding of our moral community may be a wide one, we are likely to *practise* a modified instrumentalism, sacrificing the general cause for the particular few because the general requires collective action that seems beyond our scope. I suspect these daily acts of powerlessness are psychologically hurtful. We behave, a lot of the time, as though others were means, because we do not know *how* to make them ends. The claim that this is a widespread pathology makes sense if, in thought experiment and then in action, we can reach other possible ways of being.

Samuels suggests that there is an innate desire in humans to change social and political reality (1993, p. 58). If this is the case, political indifference is pathological, the result of hurt and internal disconnection. Through better social circumstances or through psychological healing and working through, political interest and agency may be redeveloped. Samuels claims that therapy can 'fine down generalised rage into a more specific format . . . rendering emotion more accessible for social action' (1993, p. 51). My hunch is that he is right, but my evidence remains anecdotal. To get beyond it, we need studies of the psychological preconditions of effective activism and the political effects of subjectively effective therapy.

Bookchin and various green socialists ask over my shoulder what is the point in such indiscriminate psychologizing? I reply that with all respect, rationalist notions of human agency fall short on two counts. First, they skip over the question of what are rational goals, emotions and values. The answer is certainly implict in *Re-enchanting Humanity*, i.e. that while all ethics and meaning is conferred on the world and universe by human perspectives, this does not mean that, ethically speaking, 'anything goes'. Ethical and political statements about *what should be* depend on *what is*, on the nature of human beings, the world and their relationship, for evidential grounding. What human beings are like psychologically, in what conditions they suffer and thrive, is key to our choice of rational political goals – including our opposition to oppression.

Second, Bookchin and others' rationalism cannot account for collective human self-destruction. He argues that oppression interferes with awareness of reality. No doubt, but how? It is not just a matter of those in want acting according to short-term material interests rather than long-term ones. Material interests are not such obvious, psychologically given goals. People frequently cannot tell what they are or, having ascertained them, act otherwise. We need to understand the mechanisms that can make workers and management alike identify with corporate goals and understand their interests in these terms and the conditions in which they are likely to do this. Unless we theorize (in terms which are bound to be psychological) the conditions for self-deception and for awareness of reality, we are strategically and tactically hamstrung.

Deep ecology and ecofeminism are right, I believe, in their insistence that we suffer from various forms of a generalized pathology, a chronic cultural unawareness of the causes and effects of our actions. While this persists, our reparation will always be false. In our attempts to clean our sinks, we will dirty our harbours and our domestic order will remain parasitic on ecological disorder. Any healing that can increase our overall awareness of reality, of the causal chain involved in ecological destruction, of our own accountability and our corresponding power, must then be useful. To notice, as Macy advocates, how much we really care about other human beings and the natural world sounds an invaluable corrective to the defensive cynicism we breathe in with our daily greenhouse gases. But to pretend to speak for the lichen or the river at the 'Council of All Beings' is to mystify rather than to illuminate; it is to let our metaphors get dangerously out of hand.

What then of the four necessary (but not sufficient) conditions for effective ecopolitical agency?

(1)   will to change

The will to change, the inability to go on in the old way, the motivational springs to break with health-as-normal-functioning: who has these or who can acquire them in relation to ecology? For us to change the world requires a radical break with business as usual and therefore with the accepted notions of health. Potentially, everybody has it in them to change perspective, to make revolution. It has happened to the most 'unlikely' people in relation to roads' protests and protests about animal rights. In practice, how widespread this can be depends on the amount of pressure towards paradigm shift that the external world exerts (in the shape of Chernobyl and its successors), versus the addictive and comforting practices and reassurances that keep us socially conforming, with our social creativity stultified.

Who knows how much worse things will have to get, environmentally, for the balance to shift to a point when addictions and official nostrums become consciously frightening, unbelievable and anger-provoking? For each person, their group situation and individual biographies will determine not only their 'structural capacity' (Callinicos 1987, p. 87), but also their ability to use it, depending on which fears are most potent and whether glimpses of other possible ways of being can result in change. And while the will to change, to dare to put at risk the social medium of life that supports us, is one necessary ingredient to social survival, there is absolutely no guarantee that those who take that step will be able to make a realistic assessment of the situation and its needs rather than take refuge in a Messianic dream.

(2) awareness of reality

Both in the economic North and South, environmental movements are currently middle-class dominated. Dobson argues (against Porritt) that this will not always be the case, because middle-class people have more to lose, materially speaking, than the group he sees as a possible historical agent of change in Western countries at least – the unemployed (1995, p. 155). Indeed, in many countries unemployed and other marginalized people are increasingly involved in environmental campaigning, especially in direct action. But there is no reason to think the middle-class will bow out.

Ecological destruction really *is* a universal issue, as Beck claims (1992, p. 47). It does not affect everyone equally. The distribution of risk, Beck has to admit, parallels the distribution of wealth both internationally and within nations, even though it spills over on to the terrain of the economically privileged and must increasingly do so. We can expect two countervailing tendencies. On the one hand, people who feel themselves to be oppressed tend to resist. On the other, in some conditions, some forms of oppression result in denial. Ecological strategists need to study these tendencies and the social conditions in which they are expressed. For example, the daily insult of racism is often met in two broad ways. One is to defend against it in anticipation, by noting it everywhere and by expecting it so that no unrealistic hope in the oppressor group shall ever arise to be disappointed. The other is to put one's attention on similarity, not difference; to ignore racism when possible, when it cannot be ignored, to excuse it where possible, or to attribute it to a few bad members of the dominant group. I present these defensive strategies as ideal types, but in reality it is possible to vacillate between them, to mix the two or to combine either or both with a more realistic position. Each constitutes a filter on social reality, permitting awareness of some aspects and limiting it of others.

Since ecological destruction is produced by capitalist societies which also, through the same mechanisms, produce their own versions of social injustice, it *is* everybody's issue. It does not follow that everyone will be able to see it as such. Those who construe themselves as angry victims of racism, sexism, colonialism or class domination (taking the first response to oppression described above) will not be able to make common cause with the perpetrators while their own specific issues are unaddressed. Still less will they be able to identify *as* perpetrators of destruction and recognize their own active or collusive role. Their involvement with an ecological movement will only be possible if first, that movement addresses their issue, and its members who are not members of their group show themselves committed to ending that particular form of oppression. The failure of men and whites to do this convincingly is probably the reason for the dearth of women and people of colour in many Western ecological organizations. Second, they may need their own movement, which sees ecological destruction as part of the crime committed against their group, a crime which can only be forgiven when the perpetrators give up their power and make reparation. Ecofeminism is an example of this position.

For those who take the other route in response to specific social oppression (i.e. minimizing or denial), it may be more possible to *recognize* their common humanity with the oppressors and their joint status as both victims and perpetrators of the assault on the environment. Clearly there is a measure of awareness of reality here, but the denial of difference that enters the movement brings its own dangers.

It does not follow, then, that the ecologically active are more far-seeing and 'healthier' than those whose politics are focused on particular sectional interests. Middle-class people – professionals, management, small employers, non-manual service workers – are likely to be particularly sensitive to quality-of-life issues, at least for themselves (as in NIMBYism) and sometimes also for others. This is not so much because these are luxuries which only the well-off can afford, because some of the culturally middle-class – especially single parents – are poor (though there are degrees of poverty and types of work for survival which are incompatible with political campaigning).

Another reason for such concern is that the middle-class is recruited and trained via the promise of a higher quality of life for its members, in exchange for which this section of the workforce assumes responsibility for making the system work in ways which supposedly improve the overall quality of life. This is the rhetoric, suitably adapted for the various occupations. People who are often self-managing need a justificatory ideology when the systems they are concerned with seem increasingly unworkable. This large and varied group is likely to have expectations about the acceptable quality of life and about their own rights as citizens. Unsurprisingly a section of middle-class people have become environmentalists and we need not cynically assume they will never be willing to accept a reduction in their standard of living. But there is denial here, too, evidenced in the alliance between green consumerism, recycling and business-as-usual.

To put it simply, how a group is socially positioned will determine (together with more general and more specific factors) which aspect of reality its members are likely to be aware of and which they may be ignorant of or actually deny. Middle-class people are likely *both* to deny the extent of their privileges *and* the extent to which they share the situation and the material interests of other working people who are also dependent on the sale of their labour power in order to live. This is hardly surprising, since the privileges they enjoy are predicated on their separation from 'ordinary' workers and the illusion of immunity from the unacceptable aspects of employment under capitalism – such as unemployment. The way middle-class people are positioned may allow some of them to accept responsibility for environmental destruction; they are used to accepting responsibility, as the price of relative power. This does permit a sort of awareness of ecological reality, an uncomfortable assumption of guilt which may lead either to quietism or to activism. Even middle-class activists, though, may bracket the particular oppressions they share with others, as if being gay, black or female are insignificant compared with class or national privilege, and in the face of planetary threat.

I think I see this phenomenon in Macy's *World as Lover, World as Self* (1991), despite its sincere opposition to oppression and its appreciation of Buddhist philosophy. Macy is coming from a particular (and an obvious) social place, which is never acknowledged. Her language is declassed, degendered and decultured. This denial of *who the writer is* paradoxically gives it less universal appeal rather than more. She refers to Greenham Common, for instance, as a 'citizens'' rather than a 'women's' encampment, which strikes very oddly to anyone who was familiar with it. In discussing campaigns in the US she hardly ever mentions ethnic, class, generational or gender differences. This may be deliberate, but I think it a mistaken tactic.

All oppressions must be unravelled together, to permit ecopolitical agency to all. Until we recognize and claim difference and the experience of our specific oppressions, we cannot resist them effectively or work through them sufficiently to genuinely, intelligently embrace a common cause with all humanity.

(3)   movements

Perhaps coming to terms with how systematically we are lied to by governments and corporations involves feeling the terrifying disillusion that assails children when they discover how ethically shoddy, dishonest and incompetent their parents have always been. Apart from our everyday routines, our fear of the mental-health system, of looking crazy and being marginalized and disrespected, keep us cynically aloof from the goals survival requires. To be able to adopt these we need somewhere else to stand, some temporary foundation for such a radical shift of perspective, another cultural home. From such a ground we can utilize the enabling aspects of current societies, in order to break with convention and 'normal functioning' when strategically required.

An ecopolitical home must of necessity be different from dominant cultures, but it must be immanent in existing societies. To bring together the widest possible constituency, the break with normal functioning and dominant values needs clearly to emerge from ecopolitical thought and practice, so that neophytes do not have veganism and crystallography, for instance, thrust at them as obvious trappings of ecologism. It may be easier to incorporate ecological awareness into existing social-change movements and form alliances between these, than unawarely to attempt unification. If even the anti-capitalist Greens and Socialists in the UK are so culturally different that convergence (in January 1996) is difficult on these grounds alone, wider and international coalitions will take considerable time and thought.

The awareness of reality these movements need for long-term success must be fourfold. They need to hold considerable information about the actual threat and the power relations and motivations which underly destructive practices. They need to know a lot about political and economic decision-making, about the current structures, so as to be able to strategize within and against them. The need for these sorts of knowledge is generally accepted. Less recognized is the need for the following: for sociopsychological knowledge, the understanding of what can move, what upset and what paralyse people, in what situations they may unite around particular issues and how robust or fragile this unity is likely to be. Last, ecological activists need reflective knowledge of their own organizations, a way of noticing oppressive or exclusive assumptions and practices that have crept in, of loosening rigidities. 'Healing' can be an aspect of this last form of knowledge.

Healing, in the sense of recovering awareness of social and of inner reality by working through the hurtful internal effects of oppression, is necessary to the success of all ecological movements. But it need not take psychotherapeutic forms, even informal ones, any more than it need be, or ever will be 'complete'. *You Can't Kill the Spirit* (Miller, 1986) describes the development of one of the women's support groups during the British miners' strike of 1984 and how its success changed the women's relationships with their husbands, allowing them to do things of which they had never thought themselves capable. Jill Miller's book, in which women tell their own stories, shows how limited the women's expectations of life were before the strike. The women describe how miserable they were during it while still operating as individual families and how much the new culture of the support group improved their lives despite the privations. With a closeness, pride in themselves and enjoyment they envied no one. They discovered new skills in fundraising, negotiating and public speaking and new and more equal relationships with their men.

Groups can (if imaginatively run) give people authority they have nowhere else and allow their experience to be listened to with respect. They can build collegiate relationships of which many people today are completely deprived. 'It's amazing here, it's so friendly. At home, people like me get the shit kicked out of them just for what you look like,' says a young working-class boy interviewed in *The Guardian*

(13 January 1996) at the Newbury bypass protest. These experiences in movements are healing and can result in the expansion of agency, at individual and group level. The dangers are of hostility between organizations and the growth of a rigid establishment and a rigid opposition within them. Strategic and tactical thinking for ecological movements needs to study experience and theorize these dangers. On the one hand there are advantages to formal membership, which allows people to identify with an organization and allows a certain discipline and predictability. But the rigidities, abuses and limitations of party-like structures are notorious. Looser forms of organization (as at Greenham Common) can allow participants to play with possibilities, to develop their own symbolism and relationships, with the danger of the tyranny of structurelessness and the fear, for some, of being less well-contained.

(4)   human social possibilities

Finally, could human beings live in a just, ecologically sustainable society, always assuming we could overcome the enormous obstacles to building one – or would we necessarily spoil the good? There will be no final just society (though we may be living in the final, *unjust* ones). No doubt there are forms of oppression that our understanding of human beings is presently too primitive to perceive. We are only just beginning to understand the mistreatment of children. But we may well be able to build and inhabit less *dangerous* societies in which we can then face old, new and hitherto unnoticed forms of oppression and damage, and take issue with those. We have nothing to lose but our private cars, central heating and air travel. And we quite literally have a whole world to gain.

Notes

1 Her mother, a woman rejected by her husband in favour of Frau K., is also dismissed by Freud as a foolish woman, suffering from 'housewife's psychosis', who makes life 'unbearable' for everyone. Dora despises her and resents her attempt to make her daughter shoulder some responsibility for the housework. But Dora's father offers her no alternative versions of womanhood: he abandons her to the attentions of Herr K. to get peace for his own liaison.

2 Miller contends that analysis colludes with the protection of internal authority figures. She cites Freud's 1897 letter to Fliess:

> Then there was the astonishing thing that in every case blame was laid on perverse acts by the father, my own not exluded. (Freud, 1954, p. 215)

The editors, Bonaparte, Freud and Kris ommitted the words 'my own not excluded', prompting Miller's comment:

> What could have moved the editors to omit such an important phrase if not the desire to spare an internalised 'authority figure'? (1980, p. 220)

3 In 1921 Freud described society as a derivative of self-love, which became displaced, under the disillusioning criticism of parents and others, on to an 'ego-ideal'. When in later life we revere a leader or a cause, we have placed them in our ego-ideal; they become a part of ourselves which we love (1955e, p. 116). When we feel solidarity towards members of the same group, we are identifying with them because they have the same ego-ideal. Just as children accept each other's rights of access to the father on condition there is equal treatment for all, so in society:

> social justice means that we deny ourselves many things so that others may have to do without them as well . . . The demand for equality is the root of social conscience and the sense of duty. (1955e, p. 121)

4 But because it remains vague about the relationship between thinking and feeling, and the determinants of the *content* of thought, Freud's rationalism remains

sterile. For can we depend on the dominance of intellect to help us think our way out of our present dangerous situation? It was thought and science that devised and built the atom bomb; and thinking can itself be defensive – as Anna Freud recognized (1937, p. 174). To fulfil Freud's hopes in *The Future of an Illusion* the intellect would need to include the emotions within the realm of thought and to be based on human, rather than sectional interests: a distinction which Freud's reductionism in the area of sociology does not allow him to make.

5 Freud often appears to allow external events a causal role that disappears on closer examination. This can make social structures seem more influential than they actually are in his theory. Take, for instance, the sight of the genitals in the other sex, implicated in the Oedipus complex. For the boy, the sight of the girl's penis-less state lends plausibility to castration threats and leads him eventually to renounce his desire for his mother. The girl sees the boy's penis and perceives her clitoris as inferior, which eventually leads her to turn against her mother and to her father. In this account, two real events seem crucial: castration threats for the boy and for both boy and girl the sight of the genitals of the other sex. The way seems clear for social reform: stop castration threats, enlighten children about the existence of the vagina and womb, and surely the construction of gender will be affected. We might also expect differences in gender development if no sighting of the other sex's genitals occurs. Sociologists and social psychologists have gone to some lengths to show that there is no evidence for such differences (Oakley, 1981, p. 100). In fact, Freud's statements are not as empirical as they sound and in relation to castration threats he spells this out. Even if there is no father to threaten, or the father does not do so:

> children construct this danger for themselves out of the lightest hints, which will never be wanting. (1955a, p. 8)

Writing of a four-year-old whose infantile neurosis he analysed in retrospect, Freud said:

> There is no doubt whatever that at this time his father was turning into the terrifying figure that threatened him with castration ... At this point the boy has to fit himself into a phylogenetic schema, and he did so, although his personal experiences may not have agreed with it. The threats or hints of castration which he had come across had, on the contrary, emanated from women, but this could not hold up the final result for long. In spite of everything it was his father from whom in the end he came to fear castration. (1995c, p. 86)

6 The *moi* is alienated in contrast with the *je*, the 'I' of the speaking subject, but we shall see that language acquisition is itself a response to lack, i.e. to the unattainability of the object of desire. It, too, is alienated in that it marks a distancing from the immediate, wordless experience of the mirror stage. Thus each stage is alienated only in comparison with the other, not in comparison with any possible wholeness.

7 Elliott argues for a view of the unconscious as a human natural *capacity* for imaging the drives and for representation in general: 'an active accomplishment of all human agents' (Elliott, 1992, p. 28). He cites Castoriadis' critique of Lacan which argues that the imaginary is not just passive and specular, but the site of the production of images and forms (1992, p. 140).

8 In a 'true dissolution of the Oedipus complex' writes Catherine Millot in the Lacanian journal *Ornicar*, 'the demand for love . . . is rendered null and void' so that:

> the super-ego would, in Lacan's terms, be reduced to the identity of desire and law. This would correspond to Freud's post-Oedipal super-ego . . . the backbone of the subject, making him independent of all outside influence. (1985, p. 24)

This outcome, according to Millot, is rare for men but never attained by women.

9 Henriques *et al.* (1984) attempt just this by making desire historically specific, substituting historicized 'discursive relations' for Language and the timeless Symbolic order (p. 222). In Chapter 6, Cathy Urwin tries to historicize the mirror stage by suggesting that the content of the *moi* is a function of *how* the mother positions herself and is discursively positioned (p. 299). Her chapter is extremely interesting, especially in its treatment of power, but it comes much closer to object-relations theory than they would probably wish.

10 Wachtel, psychoanalyst and born-again behaviour therapist, suggests that psychoanalysis neglects the way present situations maintain the salience of the past. The behaviour involved in reaction formation, for instance, may continually feed the tendency which is being consciously denied – as when the 'nice' person, defending against childhood rage, does everything for others and continually recreates conditions for that rage. (Wachtel, 1977, p. 44)

References

AARONOWITZ, S. (1988) 'Postmodernism and Politics', in Ross, A. (Ed.) *Universal Abandon*, Minneapolis, University of Minnesota Press, pp. 47–61.

ABRAHAM, K. (1942) *Selected Papers*, London, Hogarth Press.

ALFORD, C. F. (1989) *Melanie Klein and Critical Social Theory*, New Haven, Yale University Press.

ALLEN, H. (1986) 'Psychiatry and the construction of the feminine', in MILLER, P. and ROSE N. (Eds) *The Power of Psychiatry*, Cambridge, Polity Press.

ALTHUSSER, L. (1971) *Lenin and Philosophy*, London, New Left Books.

ARCHER, M. (1995) *Realist Social Theory: the Morphogenetic Approach*, Cambridge, Cambridge University Press.

ARCHIBALD, W. P. (1989), *Marx and the Missing Link: Human Nature*, London, Macmillan.

BAKAL, D. (1979) *Psychology and Medicine*, London, Tavistock Publications.

BALINT, M. (1964) *The Doctor, his Patient and the Illness*, London, Pitman.

BALLOU, M. and GABALAC, N. W. (1985) *A Feminist Position on Mental Health*, Illinois, Thomas Books.

BANTON, R., CLIFFORD, D. P., FROSCH, S., LOUSADA, J. and ROSENTHAL, J. (1985) *The Politics of Mental Health*, London, Macmillan.

BAR, V. (1987) 'Change in women', in ERNST, S. and MAGUIRE, M. (Eds) *Living with the Sphinx*, Harmondsworth, Penguin Books.

BAUMAN, Z. (1988) 'Is there a postmodern sociology?', *Theory, Culture and Society*, 5 (2), pp. 217–39.

BAUMAN, Z. (1989a) 'Hermeneutics and Modern Social Theory', in HELD, D. and THOMPSON, J. B. (Eds) *Social Theory of Modern Societies: Anthony Giddens and his Critics*, Cambridge, Cambridge University Press, pp. 34–55.

BAUMAN, Z. (1989b) *Modernity and the Holocaust*, Cambridge, Polity Press.

BAUMAN, Z. (1990) 'From pillars to post', *Marxism Today*, February 1990.

BAVINGTON, J. (1992) 'The Bradford experiment', in KAREEM, J. and LITTLEWOOD, R. (Eds) *Intercultural Therapy*, Oxford, Blackwell.

BECK, U. (1992) *Risk Society*, London, Sage.

BENTON, E. (1989) 'Marxism and natural limits: An ecological critique and reconstruction', *New Left Review*, 178, pp. 51–86.

BERNE, E. (1975) *Transactional Analysis in Psychotherapy*, London, Souvenir Press.

BERRY, T. (1995) 'The viable human', in SESSIONS, G. (Ed.) *Deep Ecology for the Twentyfirst Century*, Boston, Shambala, pp. 8–18.

BHASKAR, R. (1975) *A Realist Theory of Science*, Leeds, Leeds Books.

BHASKAR, R. (1986) *Scientific Realism and Human Emancipation*, Hemel Hempstead, Harvester Wheatsheaf.

BHASKAR, R. (1989) *The Possibility of Naturalism*, Hemel Hempstead, Harvester Wheatsheaf.

BION, W. (1961) *Experiences in Groups*, London, Tavistock Publications.

BION, W. (1962) *Learning from Experience*, London, Heinemann.

BION, W. (1984) *Second Thoughts: Selected Papers on Psychoanalysis*, New York, Jason Aronson.

BLANCK, G. and BLANCK, R. (1974) *Ego-Psychology: Theory and Practice*, New York, Columbia University Press.

BOCK, K. (1994) *Human Nature Mythology*, Urbana and Chicago, University of Illinois Press.

BONNER, H. (1967) 'The pro-active personality', in BUGENTHAL, J. (Ed.) *Challenges in Humanistic Psychology*, New York, McGraw Hill.

BOOKCHIN, M. (1995) *Re-enchanting Humanity*, London, Cassell.

BOWIE, M. (1991) *Lacan*, London, Fontana.

BROVERMAN, I. K. (1981) 'Sex role stereotypes and clinical judgements', in HOWELL, E. and BAYES, M. (Eds) *Women and Mental Health*, New York, Basic Books.

BROWN, G. W. and HARRIS, T. (1978) *The Social Origins of Depression*, London, Tavistock Publications.

BULLARD, R. (1994) 'Environmental Racism and the Environmental Justice Movement', in MERCHANT, C. (Ed.) *Ecology*, New Jersey, Humanities Press.

BURCH, B. B. (1985) 'Another perspective on merger in lesbian relationships', in ROSEWATER, L. B. and WALKER, L. (Eds) *A Handbook of Feminist Therapy*, New York, Springer.

BUSFIELD, J. (1989) 'Sexism and psychiatry', *Sociology*, 23 (3), pp. 343–64.

CALLINICOS, A. (1987) *Making History*, Cambridge, Polity Press.

CAPRA, F. (1995) 'Deep ecology: A new paradigm', in SESSIONS, G. (Ed.) *Deep Ecology for the Twentyfirst Century*, Boston, Shambala, pp. 19–25.

CARMEN, E. H., RUSSO, N. F. and MILLER, J. B. (1984) 'Inequality and women's health', in RIEKER, P. P. and CARMEN, E. H. (Eds) *The Gender Gap in Psychotherapy*, New York, Plenum Press.

CHASSEGUET-SMIRGEL, J. and GRUNBERGER, B. (1986) *Freud or Reich?* London, Free Association Books.

CHESLER, P. (1972) *Women and Madness*, London, Allen Lane.

CHRISTIAN, J. and ISSERLIS, J. (1993) letter in *The Way Ahead*, 10.

CLARE, A. (1976) *Psychiatry in Dissent*, London, Tavistock Publications.

CLARKSON, P. (1989) *Gestalt Counselling in Action*, London, Sage.

CLEMENT, C. (1987) *The Weary Sons of Freud*, London, Verso.

COLLARD, A. (1988) *The Rape of the Wild*, London, Women's Press.

COLLIER, A. (1994) *Critical Realism*, London, Verso.

COLLINGWOOD, N. (1992) 'Deep roots of capitalism: A critique of David Wasdell's presentation on the pre and perinatal ground of capitalism and the free-market economy', unpublished paper.

COULTER, J. (1973) *Approaches to Insanity*, London, Martin Robertson.

DALY, M. (1979) *Gyn/ecology*, London, Women's Press.

D'ARDENNE, P. and MAHTANI, A. (1989) *Transcultural Counselling in Action*, London, Sage.

DE SOUSA, R. (1987) *The Rationality of Emotion*, Cambridge, Mass., MIT Press.

DINNERSTEIN, D. (1978) *The Rocking of the Cradle and the Ruling of the World*, London, Souvenir Press.

DOBSON, A. (1995) *Green Political Thought*, 2nd edn, London, Routledge.

DOYAL, L. and GOUGH, I. (1991) *A Theory of Human Need*, London, Macmillan.

DYKE, C. J. (1988) *The Evolutionary Dynamics of Complex Systems*, Oxford, Oxford University Press.

EICHENBAUM, L. and ORBACH, S. (1987) 'Separation and intimacy', in ERNST, S. and MAGUIRE, M. (Eds) *Living with the Sphinx*, Harmondsworth, Penguin Books.

ELLENBERGER, H. F. (1970) *The Discovery of the Unconscious*, New York, Basic Books.

ELLIOTT, A. (1992) *Social Theory and Psychoanalysis in Transition*, Oxford, Blackwell.

ELLIS, A. (1974) *Humanistic Psychotherapy*, New York, McGraw Hill.

ELSHTAIN, J. (1984) 'Symmetry and soporifics', in RICHARDS, B. (Ed.) *Capitalism and Infancy*, London, Free Association Books.

ELSTER, J. (1982) 'Marxism, functionalism and game theory', *Theory and Society*, 11 (4), pp. 453–82.

ERIKSON, E. (1965) *Childhood and Society*, Harmondsworth, Penguin Books.

FAIRBAIRN, R. (1952) *Psychoanalytic Studies of the Personality*, London, Routledge & Kegan Paul.

FANON, F. (1968) *Black Skin, White Masks*, London, Macgibbon & Kee.

FELMAN, S. (1987) *Jacques Lacan and the Adventure of Insight*, Cambridge Mass., Harvard University Press.

FLAX, J. (1981) 'The conflict between nurturance and autonomy in mother–daughter relations and in feminism', in HOWELL, E. and BAYES, M. (Eds) *Women and Mental Health*, New York, Basic Books.

FORRESTER, J. (1990) *The Seductions of Psychoanalysis*, Cambridge, Cambridge University Press.

FOUCAULT, M. (1967) *Madness and Civilisation*, London, Tavistock Publications.

FOUCAULT, M. (1970) *The Order of Things*, London, Routledge.

FOUCAULT, M. (1980) *Power/Knowledge*, GORDON C. (Ed.) Hemel Hempstead, Harvester.

FREUD, A. (1937) *The Ego and the Mechanisms of Defence*, London, Hogarth Press.

FREUD, A. (1966a) 'An experiment in group upbringing' (1951), in *Indications for Child Analysis and other papers 1945–56*, London, Hogarth Press.

FREUD, A. (1966b) *Normality and Pathology in Childhood*, London, Hogarth Press.

FREUD, S. (1953a) *The Interpretation of Dreams (1900)*, *Standard Edition Vols IV and V*, London, Hogarth Press.

FREUD, S. (1953b) *Three Essays on the Theory of Sexuality (1905)*, *Standard Edition Vol. VII*, London, Hogarth Press.

FREUD, S. (1953c) 'Fragment of an analysis of a case of hysteria' (1905), *Standard Edition Vol. VII*, London, Hogarth Press.

FREUD, S. (1953d) 'My views on the part played by sexuality in the aetiology of the neuroses' (1906), *Standard Edition Vol. VII*, London, Hogarth Press.

FREUD, S. (1954) 'The Origins of Psychoanalysis: Letters to William Fliess', in BONAPARTE, M., FREUD, A. and KRIS, E. (Eds) New York, Basic Books.

FREUD, S. (1955a) *Studies on Hysteria (1895)*, *Standard Edition Vol. II*, London, Hogarth Press.

FREUD, S. (1955b) 'Analysis of a phobia in a five year old boy' (1909), *Standard Edition Vol. X*, London, Hogarth Press.

FREUD, S. (1955c) 'From the history of an infantile neurosis' (1918), *Standard Edition Vol. XVII*, London, Hogarth Press.

FREUD, S. (1955d) *Beyond the Pleasure Principle (1920)*, *Standard Edition Vol. XVIII*, London, Hogarth Press.

FREUD, S. (1955e) *Group Psychology and the Analysis of the Ego (1921)*, *Standard Edition Vol. XVIII*, London, Hogarth Press.

FREUD, S. (1955f) 'Analysis terminabie and unterminable' (1937), *Standard Edition Vol. XXXIII*, London, Hogarth Press.

FREUD, S. (1955g) *An Outline of Psychoanalysis (1940)*, *Standard Edition Vol. XXIII*, London, Hogarth Press.

FREUD, S. (1957a) 'On the history of the psychoanalytic movement' (1914), *Standard Edition Vol. XIV*, London, Hogarth Press.

FREUD, S. (1957b) 'On narcissism' (1914), *Standard Edition Vol. XIV*, London, Hogarth Press.

FREUD, S. (1957c) 'Thoughts for the times on war and death' (1915), *Standard Edition Vol. XIV*, London, Hogarth Press.

FREUD, S. (1959) '"Civilised" sexual morality and modern nervous illness' (1908), *Standard Edition Vol. IX*, London, Hogarth Press.

FREUD, S. (1960) *The Psychopathology of Everyday Life (1904)*, *Standard Edition Vol. VI*, Hogarth Press, London.

FREUD, S. (1961a) *The Ego and the Id (1922)*, *Standard Edition Vol. XIX*, London, Hogarth Press.

FREUD, S. (1961b) *The Future of an Illusion (1927)*, *Standard Edition Vol. XXI*, London, Hogarth Press.

FREUD, S. (1961c) *Civilisation and its Discontents (1930)*, *Standard Edition Vol. XXI*, London, Hogarth Press.

FREUD, S. (1962a) 'Charcot' (1893) *Standard Edition Vol. III*, London, Hogarth Press.

FREUD, S. (1962b) 'The defence neuro-psychoses' (1894), *Standard Edition Vol. III*, London, Hogarth Press.

FREUD, S. (1962c) 'Heredity and the aetiology of the neuroses', *Standard Editon Vol. III*, London, Hogarth Press.

FREUD, S. (1962d) 'The aetiology of hysteria' (1896), *Standard Edition Vol. III*, London, Hogarth Press.

FREUD, S. (1962e) 'Sexuality in the aetiology of the neuroses' (1898), *Standard Edition Vol. III*, London, Hogarth Press.

FREUD, S. (1962f) 'Further remarks on the psychoneuroses of defence', *Standard Edition Vol. III*, London, Hogarth Press.

FREUD, S. (1963) *Introductory Lectures on Psychoanalysis (1916), Standard Edition Vol. XVI*, London, Hogarth Press.

FREUD, S. (1964) *New Introductory Lectures (1932), Standard Edition Vol. XXII*, London, Hogarth Press.

FROMM, E. (1971) *The Crisis in Psychoanalysis*, London, Jonathan Cape.

FROSCH, S. (1987) *The Politics of Psychoanalysis*, London, Macmillan.

FROSCH, S. (1991) *Identity Crisis*, London, Macmillan.

FUSS, D. (1989) *Essentially Speaking*, London, Routledge.

GALLOP, J. (1982) *Feminism and Psychoanalysis – The Daughter's Seduction*, London, Macmillan.

GARFINKEL, A. (1981) *Forms of Explanation*, New Haven, Yale University Press.

GEERTZ, C. (1984) 'Anti anti-relativism', *American Anthropologist*, 86, pp. 263–76.

GERAS, N. (1983) *Marx and Human Nature*, London, Verso.

GIDDENS, A. (1984) *The Constitution of Society*, Cambridge, Polity Press.

GIDDENS, A. (1990) *The Consequences of Modernity*, Cambridge, Polity Press.

GIDDENS, A. (1991) *Modernity and Self Identity*, Cambridge, Polity Press.

GLENDENNING, C. (1995) 'Recovery from Western civilisation', in SESSIONS, G. (Ed.) *Deep Ecology for the Twentyfirst Century*, Boston, Shambala, pp. 27–37.

GLOVER, E. (1945) 'An examination of the Klein system of child psychology', pamphlet reprinted from *The Psychoanalytic Study of the Child*, Vol. 1.

GOFFMAN, E. (1968) *Asylums*, Harmondsworth, Penguin Books.

GREENSPAN, M. (1983) *A New Approach to Women and Therapy*, New York, McGraw Hill.

GREY, P. (1967) 'Look at me', in SCHEFF, T. (Ed.) *Mental Illness and Social Processes*, New York, Harper & Row.

GROSSKURTH, P. (1986) *Melanie Klein*, London, Hodder & Stoughton.

GROSZ, E. (1990) *Jacques Lacan: A Feminist Introduction*, London, Routledge.

GUR, R. E., LEVY, J. and GUR, R. C. (1977) 'Clinical studies of brain organisation and behaviour', in FRAZER, A. and WINOKUR, A. (Eds) *Biological Bases of Psychiatric Disorders*, Jamaica, Spectrum.

HABERMAS, J. (1983) 'Modernity: An incomplete project', in FOSTER, H. (Ed.) *The Anti-aesthetic: Essays on Postmodernism*, Washington, Port Townsend.

HAMPDEN TURNER, C. (1970) *Radical Man: the Process of Psychosocial Development*, Cambridge Massachusetts, Schenkman Publishing Co.

HARAWAY, D. (1991) *Simians, Cyborgs and Women*, London, Free Association.

HARRIS, T. (1973) *I'm O.K. - You're O.K.*, London, Pan Books.

HARTMANN, H. (1958) *Ego Psychology and the Problem of Adaptation*, London, Imago.

HARTMANN, H. (1964) *Essays on Ego Psychology*, London, Hogarth.

HARVEY, D. (1990) *The Condition of Postmodernity*, Oxford, Blackwell.

HAYEK, F. A. (1944) *The Road to Serfdom*, London, Routledge.

HENRIQUES, J., HOLLOWAY, W., URWIN, C., VENN, C. and WALKERDINE, V. (1984) *Changing the Subject*, London, Methuen.

HERMAN, J. and HIRSCHMAN, L. (1984) 'Counselling incest survivors', in REIKER, P. P. and CARMEN, E. H. (Eds) *The Gender Gap in Psychotherapy*, New York, Plenum Press.

HINSHELWOOD, R. D. (1983) 'Projective identification and Marx's concept of man', in *The International Review of Psychoanalysis*, Vol. 10, pp. 221–5.

HINSHELWOOD, R. D. (1989) *A Dictionary of Kleinian Thought*, London, Free Association Books.

HOGGETT, P. (1992) *Partisans in an Uncertain World: The Psychoanalysis of Engagement*, London, Free Association Books.

HORNEY, K. (1937) *The Neurotic Personality of Our Time*, New York, Norton.

HOWELL, E. (1981) 'Women: from Freud to the present', in HOWELL, E. and BAYES, M. (Eds) *Women and Mental Health*, New York, Basic Books.

HUGHES, J. M. (1989) *Reshaping the Psychoanalytic Domain*, Berkeley, University of California Press.

ISAAC, J. C. (1990) 'Realism and reality: Some realistic reconsiderations', *Journal for the Theory of Social Behaviour*, 20 (1), pp. 1–31.

ISAACS, S. (1952) 'The Nature and Function of Phantasy', in KLEIN, M., HEIMANN, P., ISAACS, S. and RIVIERE, J. (Eds) *Developments in Psychoanalysis*, London, Hogarth Press, pp. 67–221.

JACKINS, H. (1965) *The Human Side of Human Beings*, Seattle, Rational Island Publishers.

JACKINS, H. (1978) *The Upward Trend*, Seattle, Rational Island Publishers.

JACKINS, H. (1981) *The Benign Reality*, Seattle, Rational Island Publishers.

JACKINS, H. (1983) *The Reclaiming of Power*, Seattle, Rational Island Publishers.

JACKINS, H. (1989) *Start Over Every Morning*, Seattle, Rational Island Publishers.

JACKINS, H. (1992) 'The chronic patterns of classism', *Present Time*, 87.

JONES, E. (1953) *Sigmund Freud: Life and Work*, Vol. III, London, Hogarth Press.

JONES, E. (1964) *The Life and Work of Sigmund Freud*, Harmondsworth, Penguin Books.

KAREEM, J. (1992) 'The NAFSIYAT Intercultural Centre', in KAREEM, J. and LITTLEWOOD, R. (Eds) *Intercultural Therapy*, Oxford, Blackwell.

KLEIN, M. (1988a) 'Symposium on child analysis' (1927), in *Love, Guilt and Reparation*, London, Virago.

KLEIN, M. (1988b) 'The importance of symbol formation in the development of the ego' (1930), in *Love, Guilt and Reparation*, London, Virago.

KLEIN, M. (1988c) 'Love, guilt and reparation' (1937), in *Love, Guilt and Reparation*, London, Virago.

KLEIN, M. (1988d) 'The Oedipus complex in the light of early anxieties' (1942), in *Love, Guilt and Reparation*, London, Virago.

KLEIN, M. (1988e) 'On observing the behaviour of young infants' (1952), in *Envy and Gratitude*, London, Virago.

KLEIN, M. (1988f) 'The psychoanalytic play technique' (1955), in *Envy and Gratitude*, London, Virago.

KLEIN, M. (1988g) 'Envy and gratitude' (1957), in *Envy and Gratitude*, London, Virago.

KORB, M. P., GORRELL, J. and VAN DE RIET, V. (1989) *Gestalt Therapy: Practice and Theory*, New York, Pergamon.

KOVEL, J. (1977) *A Complete Guide to Therapy*, Sussex, Harvester.

KOVEL, J. (1981) 'The American mental health industry', in INGLEBY, D. (Ed.) *Critical Psychiatry*, Harmondsworth, Penguin Books.

LACAN, J. (1977a) 'The mirror stage as formative of the function of the I as revealed in psychoanalytic experience' (1949), in SHERIDAN, A. (Ed.) *Ecrits: A Selection*, London, Tavistock Publications.

LACAN, J. (1977b) 'Aggressivity in psychoanalysis' (1948), in SHERIDAN, A. (Ed.) *Ecrits: A Selection*, London, Tavistock Publications.

LACAN, J. (1977c) 'Function and field of speech and language' (1953), in SHERIDAN, A. (Ed.) *Ecrits: A Selection*, London, Tavistock Publications.

LACAN, J. (1977d) 'The direction of the Treatment and the principles of its power' (1958) in SHERIDAN, A. (Ed.) *Ecrits: a Selection*, London, Tavistock.

LACAN, J. (1977e) 'The signification of the phallus', in SHERIDAN, A. (Ed.) *Ecrits: A Selection*, London, Tavistock Publications.

LACAN, J. (1979) *Four Fundamental Concepts of Psychoanalysis*, Harmondsworth, Penguin Books.

LACAN, J. and THE ECOLE FREUDIENNE (1982) *Feminine Sexuality*, MITCHELL, J. and ROSE, J. (Eds) New York, W. W. Norton.

LACAN, J. (1988a) 'The Seminar of Jacques Lacan', in MILLER, J. A. (Ed.) *Book I (1953–4)*, Cambridge, Cambridge University Press.

LACAN, J. (1988b) 'The Seminar of Jacques Lacan', in MILLER, J. A. (Ed.) *Book II (1954–5)*, Cambridge, Cambridge University Press.

LACLAU, E. and MOUFFE, C. (1985) *Hegemony and Socialist Strategy*, London, Verso.

LACLAU, E. and MOUFFE, C. (1987) 'Post-Marxism without apologies', *New Left Review*, 166, pp. 79–106.

LAING, R. D. (1960) *The Divided Self*, London, Tavistock Publications.

LAING, R. D. (1961) *Self and Others*, London, Tavistock Publications.

LANGER, M. (1989) *From Vienna to Mangua: Journey of a Psychoanalyst*, London, Free Association Books.

LAPLANCHE, J. and PONTALIS, B. (1985) *The Language of Psychoanalysis*, London, Hogarth Press.

LEE, J. SCOTT (1990) *Jacques Lacan*, Boston Mass., Twayne.

LEMAIRE, A. (1979) *Jacques Lacan*, London, Routledge & Kegan Paul.

LEMERT, C. (1992) 'General social theory, irony, postmodernism', in SEIDMAN, S.

and WAGNER, D. G. (Eds) *Postmodernism and Social Theory*, Cambridge Mass., Blackwell.

LEONARD, P. (1984) *Personality and Ideology*, London, Macmillan.

LERMAN, H. (1985) 'Some barriers to the development of a feminist theory of personality', in ROSEWATER, L. B. and WALKER, L. (Eds) *A Handbook of Feminist Therapy*, New York, Springer.

LERNER, H. (1984) 'Special issues for women in psychotherapy', in RIEKER, P. and CARMEN, E. (Eds) *The Gender Gap in Psychotherapy'*, New York, Plenum Press.

LIPSHITZ, S. (1978) '"The personal is the political": The problem of feminist therapy', in *m/f* 2, pp. 22–31.

LITTLEWOOD, R. (1990) 'From categories to contexts: A decade of the "New Cross-Cultural Psychiatry"', *British Journal of Psychiatry*, 156, pp. 308–27.

LITTLEWOOD, R. (1992) 'Towards an intercultural therapy', in KAREEM, J. and LITTLEWOOD, R. (Eds) *Intercultural Therapy*, Oxford, Blackwell.

LITTLEWOOD, R. and LIPSEDGE, M. (1981) 'Acute psychotic reactions in Caribbean-born patients', in *Psychological Medicine*, 11, pp. 303–18.

LITTLEWOOD, R. and LIPSEDGE, M. (1989) *Aliens and Alienists*, London, Unwin Hyman.

LOVE, B. (1994) 'Healing the hurts of racism: Guidelines for allies', unpublished pamphlet.

MACY, J. (1991) *World as Lover, World as Self*, Berkeley, Parallax Press.

McGOVERN, D. and COPE, R. V. (1987) 'The compulsory detention of males of different ethnic groups', *British Journal of Psychiatry*, 150, pp. 505–12.

McGRATH, W. (1986) *Freud's Discovery of Psychoanalysis: The Politics of Hysteria*, Ithaca, Cornell University Press.

MAGUIRE, M. (1987) 'Casting the evil eye', in ERNST, S. and MAGUIRE, M. (Eds) *Living with the Sphinx*, Harmondsworth, Penguin Books.

MALCOLM, J. (1984) *In the Freud Archives*, London, Jonthan Cape.

MALINOWSKI, B. (1960) *Sex and Repression in Savage Society*, London, Routledge & Kegan Paul.

MANNONI, O. (1971) *Freud: The Theory of the Unconscious*, London, New Left Books.

MARCUSE, H. (1972) *Eros and Civilisation*, London, Abacus.

MARSELLA, A. J. and WHITE, G. M. (Eds) (1982) *Cultural Conceptions of Mental Health and Therapy*, London, D. Reidel.

MARX, K. (1966) *Das Kapital, Volume III*, Moscow, Progress Publishers.

MASLOW, A. (1968) *Towards a Psychology of Being*, New York, D. Van Nostrand.

MASLOW, A. (1973) *The Farther Reaches of Human Nature*, Harmondsworth, Penguin Books.

MASLOW, A. (1976) *Religion, Values and Peak-Experiences*, Harmondsworth, Penguin Books.

MASSON, J. (1984) *Freud: The Assault on Truth*, London, Faber & Faber.

MELLOR, M. (1992) *Breaking the Boundaries: Towards a Feminist Green Socialism*, London, Virago.

MENZIES-LYTH, I. (1988) *Containing Anxiety in Institutions, Selected Essays Vol. I*, London, Free Association Books.

MERCER, K. (1986) 'Racism and transcultural psychiatry', in MILLER, P. and ROSE, N. (Eds) *The Power of Psychiatry*, Cambridge, Polity Press.

MILLER, A. (1983) *The Drama of the Gifted Child*, London, Virago.

MILLER, A. (1985) *Thou Shalt Not Be Aware*, London, Pluto Press.

MILLER, J. (1986) *You Can't Kill the Spirit*, London, The Women's Press.

MILLER, J. B. (1978) *Towards a New Psychology of Women*, Harmondsworth, Penguin Books.

MILLER, J. B. (1984) 'The effect of inequality on psychology', in REITER, P. and CARMEN, E. (Eds) *The Gender Gap in Psychotherapy*, New York, Plenum Press.

MILLETT, K. (1991) *The Loony Bin Trip*, London, Virago.

MILLIGAN, D. (1980) *Reasoning and the Explanation of Actions*, Sussex, Harvester Press.

MILLOT, C. (1985) 'The feminine super-ego', *m/f*, 10.

MITCHELL, J. (1975) *Psychoanalysis and Feminism*, Harmondsworth, Penguin Books.

MONEY-KYRLE, R. R. (1944) 'Aspects of political ethics from the psychoanalytic point of view', *International Journal of Psychoanalysis*, Vol. XXV, 3, pp. 166–71.

MONEY-KYRLE, R. R. (1952) 'Psychoanalysis and ethics', *International Journal of Psychoanalysis*, Vol. XXXIII, 2, pp. 225–34.

NAESS, A. (1995a) 'The deep ecological movement', in SESSIONS, G. (Ed.) *Deep Ecology for the Twentyfirst Century*, Boston, Shambala, pp. 64–84.

NAESS, A. (1995b) 'Equality, sameness and rights', in SESSIONS, G. (Ed.) *Deep Ecology for the Twentyfirst Century*, Boston, Shambala, pp. 222–4.

NAESS, A. (1995c) 'Self-realisation: An ecological approach to being in the world', in SESSIONS, G. (Ed.) *Deep Ecology for the Twentyfirst Century*, Boston, Shambala, pp. 225–39.

NAESS, A. (1995d) 'The Third World, wilderness and deep ecology', in SESSIONS, G. (Ed.) *Deep Ecology for the Twentyfirst Century*, Boston, Shambala, pp. 397–407.

NARANJO, C. (1972) 'Present-centredness: Technique, prescription and ideal', in FAGAN, J. and SHEPHERD, I. (Eds) *Gestalt Therapy Now*, Harmondsworth, Penguin Books.

NEW, C. (1994) 'Structure, agency and social transformation', *Journal for the Theory of Social Behaviour*, 24 (3), pp. 187–205.

OAKLEY, A. (1981) *Subject Woman*, Oxford, Martin Robertson.

OPLER, M. K. (1969) 'Anthropological contributions to psychiatry and social psychology', in PLOG, S. C. and EDGERTON, R. B. (Eds) *Changing Perspectives in Mental Illness*, New York, Holt, Rinehart & Winston.

PEPPER, D. (1993) *Eco-Socialism: From Deep Ecology to Social Justice*, London, Routledge.

PERLS, F. S. (1972) 'Four lectures', in FAGAN, J. and SHEPHERD, I. (Eds) *Gestalt Therapy Now*, Harmondsworth, Penguin Books.

PERLS, F. S., HEFFERLINE, R. F. and GOODMAN, P. (1951) *Gestalt Therapy*, London, Souvenir Press.

PERLS, L. (1972) 'One Gestalt therapist's approach', in FAGAN, J. and SHEPHERD, I. (Eds) *Gestalt Therapy Now*, Harmondsworth, Penguin Books.

PILGRIM, D. and ROGERS, A. (1993) *A Sociology of Mental Health and Illness*, Buckingham, Open University Press.

PLANT, J. (Ed.) (1989) *Healing the Wounds: The Promise of Ecofeminism*, Philadelphia, New Society Publishers.

PLECK, J. H. (1984) 'Men's power with women, other men and society', in RIEKER, P. P. and CARMEN, E. H. (Eds) *The Gender Gap in Psychotherapy*, New York, Plenum Press.

PLUMWOOD, V. (1993) *Feminism and the Mastery of Nature*, London, Routledge.

RED-GREEN STUDY GROUP (1995) *What on Earth Is To Be Done?* Manchester.

REICH, W. (1951) *The Sexual Revolution*, London, Vision Press.

REICH, W. (1968) *The Function of the Orgasm*, London, Panther.

RIEKER, P. and CARMEN, E. (1984) *The Gender Gap in Psychotherapy*, New York, Plenum Press.

ROGERS, C. (1990) *The Carl Rogers Reader*, London, Constable.

RORTY, R. (1979) *Philosophy and the Mirror of Nature*, Princeton, Princeton University Press.

ROSE, J. (1982) 'Introduction II', in LACAN, J. and the Ecole Freudienne, *Feminine Sexuality*, MITCHELL, J. and ROSE, J. (Eds), London, Macmillan, pp. 27–57.

ROUSTANG, F. (1990) *The Lacanian Delusion*, Oxford, Oxford University Press.

ROWAN, J. (1988) *Ordinary Ecstasy*, London, Routledge.

ROWE, D. (1985) *Living with the Bomb*, London, Routledge & Kegan Paul.

RUSTIN, M. (1991) *The Good Society and the Inner World*, London, Verso.

RYCROFT, C. (1984) 'A case of hysteria', *The New York Review*, 12 April 1984.

SACHS, W. (1993) *Global Ecology*, London, Zed Books.

SACKS, O. (1982) *Awakenings*, Harmondsworth, Penguin Books.

SAFOUAN, M. (1981) 'Is the Oedipus complex universal?' *m/f*, 5/6, pp. 83–90.

SAMUELS, A. (1993) *The Political Psyche*, London, Routledge.

SAYER, A. (1992) *Method in Social Science*, London, Routledge.

SAYERS, J. (1991) *Mothering Psychoanalysis*, London, Hamish Hamilton.

SAYERS, S. (1989) 'Work, leisure and human needs', in WINNIFRITH, T. and BARRETT, C. (Eds) *The Philosophy of Leisure*, London, Macmillan.

SAYERS, S. (1990) 'Marxism and actually existing socialism', in MCLELLAN, D. and SAYERS, S. (Eds) *Socialism and Morality*, London, Macmillan.

SCHELL, J. (1982) *The Fate of the Earth*, London, Picador.

SCHNEIDERMAN, S. (1983) *Jacques Lacan – the Death of an Intellectual Hero*, Cambridge Mass., Harvard University Press.

SCOTT, A. (1988) 'Feminism and the seductiveness of the "real event"', *Feminist Review*, 28, pp. 88–102.

SEAGER, J. (1993) *Earth Follies: Feminism, Politics and the Environment*, London, Earthscan.

SEDGEWICK, P. (1982) *Psychopolitics*, London, Pluto Press.

SEGAL, H. (1964) *Introduction to the Work of Melanie Klein*, London, Heinemann.

SEGAL, H. (1987) 'Silence is the real crime', *The International Review of Psychoanalysis*, 14 (3), pp. 3–10.

SEIDMAN, S. (1992) 'Theory as narrative with moral intent', in SEIDMAN, S. and WAGNER, D. G. (Eds) *Postmodernism and Social Theory*, Cambridge Mass., Blackwell.

SESSIONS, G. (Ed.) (1995) *Deep Ecology for the Twentyfirst Century*, Boston, Shambala.

SHEPARD, P. (1995) 'Ecology and man – a viewpoint', in SESSIONS, G. (Ed.) *Deep Ecology for the Twentyfirst Century*, Boston, Shambala, pp. 131–40.

SHIVA, V. (1989) 'Development, ecology and women', in PLANT, J. (Ed.) *Healing the Wounds: the Promise of Ecofeminism*, Philadelphia, New Society Publishers.

SHOWALTER, E. (1987) *The Female Malady*, London, Virago.

SIEGEL, R. J. (1983) 'Change and creativity at midlife', in ROBBINS, J. H. and SIEGEL, R. J. (Eds) *Women Changing Therapy*, New York, Haworth Press.

SIEGLER, M. and OSMOND, H. (1976) *Models of Madness, Models of Medicine*, New York, Macmillan.

SMITH, A. J. and SIEGEL, R. J. (1985) 'Redefining power for the powerless', in ROSEWATER, L. B. and WALKER, L. W. (Eds) *A Handbook of Feminist Therapy*, New York, Springer.

SMITH, D. (1978) 'K. is mentally ill', *Sociology*, 12 (1), pp. 23–53.

SNYDER, G. (1995) 'Cultured or crabbed', in SESSIONS, G. (Ed.) *Deep Ecology for the Twentyfirst Century*, Boston, Shambala, pp. 47–9.

SOPER, K. (1981) *On Human Need*, Brighton, Harvester.

STACEY, M. (1976) 'Concepts of health and illness', SSRC Working Paper.

STARHAWK, (1989) 'Feminist, earth-based spirituality and ecofeminism', in PLANT, J. (Ed.) *Healing the Wounds: The Promise of Ecofeminism*, Philadelphia, New Society Publishers, pp. 174–85.

STURDIVANT, S. (1980) *Treatment with Women, A Feminist Philosophy of Treatment*, New York, Springer.

SUE, D. W. and SUE, D. (1981) *Counselling the Culturally Different*, New York, Wiley.

SULLIVAN, H. S. (1964) *The Fusion of Psychiatry and Social Science*, New York, W. W. Norton.

SYMINGTON, N. (1986) *The Analytic Experience*, London, Free Association Books.

SZASZ, T. (1974) *Law, Liberty and Psychiatry*, London, Routledge.

SZASZ, T. (1976) *The Myth of Mental Illness*, New York, Harper & Row.

THOMAS, C. S. and COMER, J. P. (1973) 'Racism and mental health services', in WILLIE, C. V., KRAMER, B. M. and BROWN, B. S. (Eds) *Racism and Mental Health*, Pittsburgh, University of Pittsburgh Press.

THOMAS, L. (1992) 'Working with racism in the consulting room: An Analytic View', in KAREEM, J. and LITTLEWOOD, R. (Eds) *Intercultural Therapy*, Oxford, Blackwell.

TURKLE, S. (1979) *Psychoanalytic Politics*, London, Burnett Books.

VAN DER LEEUW, (1971) 'On the development of the concept of defence', *International Journal of Psychoanalysis*, 52, pp. 51–8.

VEITH, I. (1965) *Hysteria: The History of a Disease*, Chicago, University of Chicago Press.

WACHTEL, P. L. (1977) *Psychoanalysis and Behaviour Therapy*, New York, Basic Books.

WASDELL, D. (1989) 'Constraints encountered in the conduct of psycho-social analysis', CONNECT, Paper No. 8.

WILCOX, P. (1973) 'Positive mental health in the black community', in WILLIE, C. V., KRAMER, B. M. and BROWN, B. S. (Eds) *Racism and Mental Health*, Pittsburgh, University of Pittsburgh Press.

WINNICOTT, D. (1971) *Playing and Reality* (2nd Edition), London, Tavistock Publications.

WORLD COMMISSION ON ENVIRONMENT AND DEVELOPMENT, (1987) *Our Common Future*, Oxford, Oxford University Press.

WRIGHT, W. (1982) *The Social Logic of Health*, New Brunswick, Rutgers University Press.

YOUNG-BRUEHL, E. (1988) *Anna Freud*, New York, Summit Books.

Index

Aaronowitz, S. 5
Abraham, K. 56, 70
action 21, 23, 104
  causes of 29, 105, 115–16
  and health 35, 37
  political 4, 44, 122, 129–30, 133, 141,
    149
  rational social 97, 102, 106, 156
  transformative 2, 24, 42, 143
adjustment, as criterion of health 40, 63–5,
  104, 129, 131
agency 144
  constraints on 15, 21, 77, 85–6
  ecological 143–59
  health and 29–31, 38
  rational 47, 64, 97, 102
  scepticism about 2, 20, 87, 90, 97,
    102
  theories of 20–5, 115–16, 119–22
agents
  free 27
  knowledgeable 22
  moral 27
  rational 102
Alford, C. F. 70, 73, 82–3
alienation 78, 84, 91, 105
Allen, H. 130
Althusser, L. 87–8
anger, righteous 43, 57, 86, 108, 121, 123,
  129–30
anthropocentrism 14, 16, 17
Archer, M. 23
Archibald, W. P. 20

Backal, D. 31, 33
Balint, M. 32
Ballou, M. and Gabalac, N. W. 125, 131
Banton, R. 99–100, 101
Bar, V. 127
Bauman, Z. 4, 5, 43
Bavington, J. 132
Beck, U. 5, 163
Benton, T. 6, 18
Berry, T. 154
Bhaskar, R. 6, 7, 8, 20–2, 26, 28
  transformational model of social activity
    21–3
Bion, W. 78, 83–4, 128
Blanck, G. and Blanck, R. 65
Blanck, R., see Blanck, G.
Bock, K. 144
Bookchin, M. 152–4, 162
Bowie, M. 94, 95
Broverman, I. K. 128, 130
Brown, G. and Harris, T. 131–2
Brundtland report 12, 15–16, 151
  see also World Commission on
    Environment and Development
Bullard, R. 150
business as usual 156, 163, 165
  see also health as normal functioning

Callinicos, A. 25, 163
capitalism 16–18, 82, 141, 152–3, 164
Capra, F. 155
Carmen, E. H., Russo, N. F. and Miller,
  J. B. 131

castration 53, 66, 72, 98, 169
  threats of 59, 68, 93, 96
causally generative mechanisms 19, 42
Charcot, J. M. 49
Chasseguet-Smirgel, J. 134
  and Grunberger, B. 119, 121
Chesler, P. 34, 131
Clare, A. 32
Clarkson, P. 108, 110
class 17, 20, 67, 117, 133, 137–8, 140,
  163
Clement, C. 87, 88, 96
co-counselling *see* Re-evaluation
  Counselling
Collard, A. 158
Collier, A. 6, 28
Collingwood, N. 140–1
Comer, J. P. *see* Thomas, C. S. and
  Comer, J. P.
CONNECT 140–1
consciousness raising 124
constitutional differences 46, 53, 54, 74,
  79
construction of subjectivity 149
Controversial Discussions 70–1
Cope, R. V. 127
Coulter, J. 34
critical realism 6–8, 34, 37, 114, 139

D'Ardenne, P. and Mahtani, A. 128
Daly, M. 41
death instinct 47, 58–9, 71, 73–4, 76, 78,
  82
deep ecology 13, 16, 18, 66, 145, 154–7,
  159, 162
deficit models 131, 133–4, 136, 139–40,
  141, 149
denial
  of danger 9, 82–3
  as defence 39–42, 44, 63, 80, 82–3,
    113, 117, 155
  humanistic explanations 113, 117, 160
depressive position 74, 76, 81, 83
De Sousa, R. 36, 41
Dinnerstein, D. 85

discourse determinism 90
  see also linguistic idealism
dissipative structures 13
Dobson, A. 18, 157
Doyal, L. and Gough, I. 15, 20, 135
dualism
  deconstruction of 158–9
  individual/society 71, 90, 138
  mind/body 31–2
Dyke, C. J. 13, 18, 20
  *Evolutionary Dynamics of Complex
    Systems, The* 13
  'pathways through the possible' 20

Earth First! 159
ecocentrism 14, 154
ecofeminism 41, 85, 116, 142, 157–9, 162
  differences between 157–8
Ecole Française de Paris 88
Ecole Freudienne 89
ecological destruction *see* environmental
  destruction
ecological sustainability 17, 42, 143, 150
ego
  in ego psychology 62–6, 103
  in Freud 57–60
  in Klein 72–4
  in Lacan 87, 91, 97, 102, 103
ego psychology 62–6, 102, 103–4, 145
Eichenbaum, L. and Orbach, S. 127
  see also Orbach, S. and Eichenbaum, L.
Ellenberger, H. F. 46, 47, 48
Elliott, A. 93, 95
Ellis, A. 106
Elster, J. 26
emancipation 3–8, 10, 28
embodiment 19, 29
empiricism 125
  anti-empiricism 1
environmental destruction 13, 14, 38–40,
  141, 154–5, 162, 164–5
environmental threat 7, 9–10, 12, 15, 17
  responses to 39–40, 47, 62, 68, 83, 86,
    102, 143, 166
environmentalism 12–16, 151

epistemology 3, 4
evolutionary theory 61, 108, 144
existential psychotherapy 105
existentialism 105

Fairbairn, R. 71, 75, 103
Fanon, F. 129
fantasy 53, 55–7
  see also phantasy
feminist therapy 124–32
Ferenczi, S. 61, 70, 121
Flax, J. 127
Fliess, W. 47, 50, 52
Foucault, M. 3, 4, 7, 31
Freud, A. 47, 62–6, 70–2, 81, 88, 97
  *The Ego and the Mechanisms of
    Defence* 62
Freud, S. 33, 40–1, 46–69, 81, 92, 98,
  145–6
  Analysis Terminable and Interminable
    98
  Beyond the Pleasure Principle 47, 58,
    59
  causal role of external factors 49, 51–2,
    54–5, 66–8, 169
  causal role of intra-psychic factors 52–3,
    54
  Civilisation and its Discontents 60, 153
  Dora 56
  ego 57–60, 65–6, 97
  Ego and the Id, The 47, 59
  Future of an Illusion, The 67, 153
  health and illness 46–7, 48, 51, 54, 60
  Interpretation of Dreams, The 40, 47,
    52, 53, 87
  Little Hans 54, 67
  mental health 52, 58, 62, 65–6
  Oedipus 53, 59
  'On Narcissism' 47, 57, 58
  *On the History of the Psychoanalytical
    Movement* 55
  phylogenesis 92–3
  Psychopathology of Everyday Life, The
    53
  rationality 47, 61

repression 41, 52, 57–9
Studies in Hysteria 50
superiority of penis 93
Three Essays on the Theory of Sexuality
  53, 58
trauma theory 49–5, 56
unconscious, the 47, 53, 61
Fromm, E. 47, 103
Frosch, S. 10, 74, 87, 90, 93, 103, 114,
  136

Gabalac, N. W. *see* Ballou, M. and
  Gabalac, N. W.
Gallop, J. 94, 101
Garfinkel, A. 20
Geertz, C. 138–9
Geras, N. 20
Gestalt 107, 109, 113, 115–16
  prayer 110
Giddens, A. 5, 6, 21–3, 39
  Modernity and Self Identity 22
  structuration theory 21–3
Glendenning, C. 155
Glover, E. 71–2
Goffman, E. 36
Goodman, P. 108
Gough, I. *see* Doyal, L. and Gough, I.
Greenspan, M. 127, 130
Grey, P. 34
Gorrell, J. *see* Korb, M. P. *et al.*
Grosskurth, P. 71
Grosz, E. 99
Grunberger, B. *see* Chasseguet-Smirgel, J.
  and Grunberger, B.
Guntrip, H. 71, 75, 103

Habermas, J. 3
Hampden-Turner, C. 113
Haraway, D. 4
Harris, T. 104
Hartmann, H. 63–5, 81
  *Ego Psychology and the Problem of
    Adaptation* 64
Harvey, D. 4
Hayek, F. A. 43

health
  gendered 126, 131
  mental health 28, 41, 108, 128
  normal functioning 30, 37–42, 64–5, 80,
      124, 142, 143, 156, 161–2
  positive health 37, 40–3, 104, 106,
      111–13, 132–3, 143, 160, 161
  social health 123, 141
  as state of full humanness 30
Hefferline, R. F. 108
Henriques, J., Holloway, W., Urwin, C.,
      Venn, C. and Walkerdine, V. 87,
      90
heterosexuality 22, 48, 53, 58, 85, 121
Hinshelwood, R. 71, 72, 73, 74, 76, 77,
      78
history
  human capacity to make 23–5, 77
Hoggett, P. 41, 43, 77, 83, 146–7
Holloway, W. *see* Henriques, J. *et al.*
homosexuality 57, 121
Horney, K. 99, 103, 133
Howell, E. 131
Hughes, J. M. 73
human capacities 108
human nature 9, 14, 15, 107, 139
  and denial 41–2, 44, 115
  physical 19
  potential of 110
  psychological 19–20, 22, 42–4, 46
    in humanistic psychology 106, 114
    in Lacan 96, 99–101, 102
human needs 14–15, 41, 88, 107, 108
  basic 14, 15, 35, 110, 135
  effect if unmet 108, 135–6, 160
  Maslow's theory 110
  in RC 135–6
humanism 14
  anti-humanism 87
humanistic psychology 147–8
  causal role of external factors 113–18
  general characteristics 104–6
  notions of health 103, 108, 111–13
  and psychoanalysis 103–4, 108, 109,
      111, 115, 121–2

illness 30–6
  mental illness 32–7
interests 25–6, 27, 28
internal objects 72–4
Isaacs, S. 71–2

Jackins, H. 134–8
Jacques, E. 79
Jones, E. 46, 53, 61

Kareem, J. 128
Kernberg, O. 103
Klein, M. 70–84, 127, 146–7
  causal role of external factors 73–7
  death instinct 73, 74–6, 86
  depressive position 74, 76, 81
  envy 74–5, 84, 144
  epistemophilia 76
  gender, account of 84–5
  internal objects 72–4
  Oedipus 72
  paranoid-schizoid stage 74, 76
  phantasy 71–2, 79
  projective identification 78–9
  psychological health 80–4, 120
  reparation 81–2, 84, 86, 130, 146
knowledge 3, 7, 8, 37, 126
  adequacy of 144
  flight from 83–4
  foundations 3, 98
  in Klein 71, 84
  local 3–6
  women's 125, 159
Kohut, H. 103
Korb, M. P., Gorrell, J., and Van de Riet,
      V. 109, 110
Kovel, J. 34, 104, 122

labelling theory 33, 131
Lacan, J. 87–102, 119, 121
  castration 98, 99, 102
  causal role of external factors 92, 99,
      100–1
  desire 95–6, 98, 102
  ego 87, 91, 97, 102, 103

on Freud, A. 97
goal of analysis 89, 96–8, 98
Imaginary, the 91, 100
jouissance 98
on Klein 101
Language 91–2, 94, 96, 99, 100
Law of the Father 92, 101
mirror stage 88, 91, 95, 100
objets petit a 94–5
Oedipus 91–2, 93, 94, 96
pass, the 89
phallus 92–5, 99
political position 88–9
real, the 93, 94, 100
seminars 88–9, 90, 98
sexual difference 95, 98
Symbolic, the 91, 94, 100
Laclau, E. and Mouffe, C. 4, 5
Laing, R. 38, 105, 128
Langer, M. 124
Lee, S. 99
Lemaire, A. 93
Lemert, C. 3
Leonard, P. 38
Lerman, H. 132
Lerner, H. 127, 128, 129
levels of reality 20
Levy, J. 29
linguistic idealism 100
    see also discourse determinism
Lipschitz, S. 125, 127
Littlewood, R. 127, 132
    and Lipsedge, M. 127, 128, 132–3

McGovern, D. 127
McGrath, W. 54
Macy, J. 156, 162, 165
Maguire, M. 134
Mahtani, A. *see* D'Ardenne, P. and
    Mahtani, A.
Malcolm, J. 120
Malinowski, B. 127
Mannoni, O. 64
Marcuse, H. 58
Marsella, A. J. 34

Marx, K. 8, 20, 68
Marxism 17–18, 19
Maslow, A. 105–7, 109–15, 118, 148
    B-cognisers *see* self-actualization
    self-actualization 111–13, 115, 118, 160
    theory of needs 110–11, 148–9
Masson, J. 47, 54
medical model 31, 34, 96, 105–6
Mellor, M. 157
mental illness 31, 32, 51, 60
    and physical illness 32
    real states involved 34
Menzies Lyth 79–80, 84
Mercer, K. 127, 132
Miller, A. 47, 54, 56, 135, 168
Miller, J. 166
Miller, J. B. 132
Millett, K. 33
Millot, C. 170
Mitchell, J. 94
modernity 3–4, 16
Money Kyrle, R. R. 81–2
motivation 19, 22, 25, 27, 42, 47, 111
    for ecological activism 143, 145, 146,
        148, 151, 153, 166
movements, social 5, 9, 10, 43, 81, 118,
        125, 143–53, 157–67

Naess, A. 14, 17, 155
Naranjo, C. 110, 113
needs, *see* human needs

objects, internal 72–4
object relations theory 71, 75, 76, 78–9,
        91, 103, 136, 170
Oedipus 53, 59, 72, 91–2, 93, 94, 96, 127
Ogden, T. 74
Opler, M. K. 179
oppression 129, 130–2, 136, 149, 162,
        164, 167
    internalized oppression 117, 139
Orbach, S. and Eichenbaum, L. 134
    see also Eichenbaum, L. and Orbach, S.
Osmond, H. *see* Siegler, M. and Osmond,
    H.

paranoid schizoid position 74, 76
peak experiences 104
Pepper, D. 17
Perls, F. 107, 109–10, 112, 115
person centered counselling *see* Rogers
phallus 92–3, 99
phantasy 71–2, 79
    see also fantasy
phenomenology 96, 105
Plant, J. 158
Pleck, J. 134
Plumwood, V. 158, 160–1
    relational self 160–2
postmodernism 19
poststructuralism 4, 19
psychoanalysis
    and humanistic psychology 121–2
    and sexual difference 59, 85, 98, 99
    therapeutic aims 88–9, 98, 129
    transference 70, 104, 127–8
psychological health 34, 40, 130
    in Anna Freud 63–4
    in deep ecology 155–6
    in feminist therapy 131–4
    in Freud 52, 58, 62
    in humanistic psychology 104, 109–11
    in Klein 80–4
    in Lacan 96
    in transcultural therapy 132–4
psychological structures 2, 27, 44–5
    in Freud 66–7
    in Klein 76–7
    in Lacan 100
    relationship to social 113–14, 118, 129, 139, 141
psychology 19–20, 25–7
'Psychotherapists and Counsellors for Social Responsibility' 122

racism 37, 43, 61, 77, 79, 117
    environmental 150
    Re-evaluation Counselling view 137–8
    transcultural therapy view 124, 132–4
radical social change, conditions for 25, 42–3, 143–4

rational choice theory 26
rational emotive therapy 106
rationalization 85
Red-Green Study Group 14
reductionism 29, 119, 131, 169
Re-evaluation Counselling 134–41
    distress patterns 135–6
    Present Time 134
    theory of oppression 137–8
reflexivity 24, 42–3, 147, 166
Reich, W. 58, 103, 119
relativism 7, 8, 34, 64, 133
reparation 81–2, 84, 86, 146, 155, 162
repression
    in Freud 41, 52, 54, 56–9
    in Lacan 101
Rieker, P. P. and Carmen, E. H. 131
risk 142, 163
Rogers, C. 106–7, 110, 116–17, 148
    fully functioning person 111
    unconditional positive regard 109
    wisdom of the organism 108, 128
Rorty, R. 8
Rose, J. 94, 98
Roustang, F. 88, 90
Rowan, J. 116, 117–18
Rowe, D. 39, 150–1
Rustin, M. 78, 79, 81, 82, 147

Sachs, W. 17
Sacks, O. 38
Safouan, M. 92
Samuels, A. 78–9, 122–3, 155, 161
Sayer, A. 4, 7
Sayers, J. 91
Sayers, S. 15
Saussure, S. 93
Schell, J. 16, 41
Schneiderman, S. 89, 96, 98, 102
Scott, A. 55
Seager, J. 142
Sedgewick, P. 30
seduction theory *see* Freud, trauma theory
Segal, H. 73, 81, 83, 122
Seidman, S. 3

self
  construction of 85, 103, 113, 120, 129,
    132
  ecological 155, 161
  real 110, 114
  relational 160–2
  true 64, 68, 103, 138, 139
self-actualization *see* Maslow
Sessions, G. 12, 17
Shiva, V. 158
Showalter, E. 34, 48
Siegel, R. J. 126
Siegler, M. and Osmond, H. 30
Smith, A. J. 126
Smith, D. 33
Snyder, G. 155
social constructionism 99
social defence systems 79–80, 83
social ecology 148, 152–4
social structures 21, 23–5, 44–5, 137,
    141
  causal role of 54, 119–20
  in humanistic psychology 115, 117
  in Klein 76–7, 80
  in Lacan 100
  relationship to psychological 113–14,
    118, 129, 139, 141
social transformation 2, 22, 143
socialism 1, 2, 4, 9, 17–18, 43, 81, 124,
    154
Société Française de Psychoanalyse 88
Soper, K. 6, 15–16
Stacey, M. 37
Starhawk, 158
structural capacities 25, 163
structural changes 22–5, 117
structuralism 20, 89–90
Sturdivant, S. 128
subject 2, 74, 154
  construction in Language 87, 90,
    101–2
  embodied 19–20, 29
  illusory 97, 119
Sue, D. W. and Sue, D. 128
Sullivan, H. S. 103

sustainable development 13, 15, 17
Sutich, A. J. 106
Symington, N. 46
synergy 107, 118
Szasz, T. 115

Tavistock Institute 79
therapy
  existential 105
  feminist 124–32
  'for the world' 140, 142
  politics of 128–30
  psychoanalytic *see* Freud, Klein, Lacan
  rational-emotive 106
  transcultural 124, 127–34
Thomas, C. S. and Comer, J. P. 128
Thomas, L. 129, 132
Transactional Analysis 104, 121
Transcultural Psychiatry Society 127
transcultural therapy 124, 127–34
transference 70, 104, 127–8
  social 140
Turkle, S. 88, 89, 99

unconscious
  constraints on agency 61, 85, 119, 127
  fantasy 53, 55–7
  in humanistic psychology 111, 112, 115,
    116
  and intentionality 32, 47, 115–16
  in Lacan 88, 93, 95, 97, 100–2
  meaning of environmental damage
    10
  phantasy 71–2, 79
  pleasure principle in 40, 53
  role in health 58, 111, 119, 129
  whether socially influenced 121, 123
  wishes 70
unintended consequences 5, 16, 21, 23,
    25
Urwin, C. *see* Henriques, J. *et al.*

Van de Riet, V. *see* Korb *et al.*
Van der Leeuw, A. 65
Veith, I. 48

Venn, C. *see* Henriques, J. *et al.*
voluntarism 21, 89, 115, 126

Wachtel, P. 170
Walkerdine, V. *see* Henriques, J. *et al.*
Wasdell, D. 140–1
White, G. N. 34
Wilcox, P. 134

Winnicott, D. 75, 81, 85, 103, 147
World Commission on Environment and
  Development 12, 15, 17
  Our Common Future 13
World Health Organisation 37
Wright, W. 30, 34

Young-Bruehl, E. 72